FITACTIONS

NO B.S. TAKE ACTION FITNESS

, HABITS AND HACKS FOR MEN

TO PACK ON MUSCLE, BOOST ENERGY and
LIVE FIT, FOREVER!

"Reading is for your mind.
Fit Actions was written for
results! Take action today and
see results tomorrow!"

-Doug Bennett

The problem with most fitness and diet books is that they fill up the pages with lots of copycat information, without giving direct action steps to getting results. Doug Bennett, at 50 years old and still wrestling division 1A college athletes has decided to change all that. He has written a laser focused, <u>Take Action Book</u> called *Fit Actions* to help guys after 35 increase their fitness level, energy, metabolism and to be a strong, fit man.

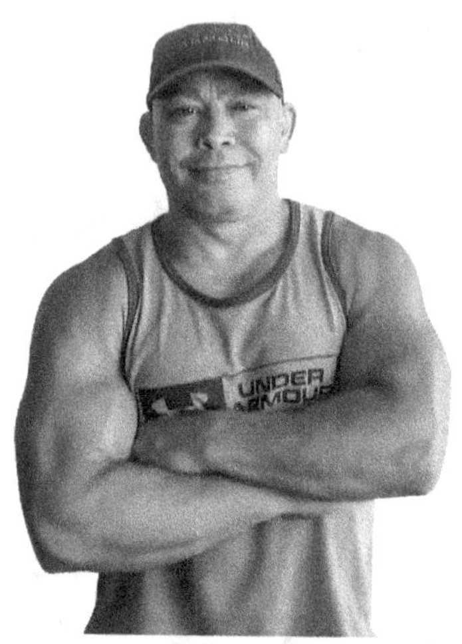

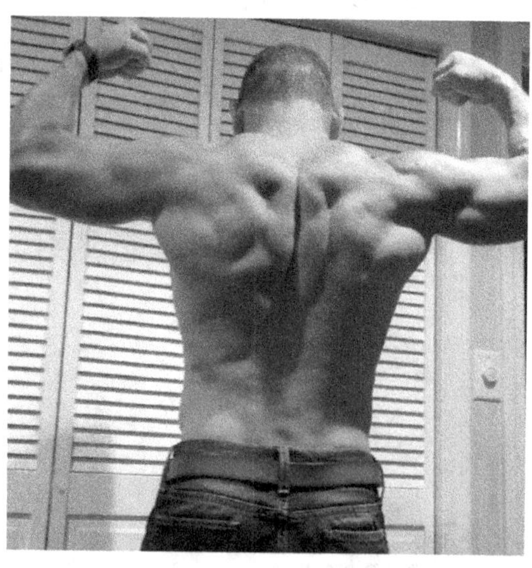

Table of Contents

Why I Wrote This Book:

Look, I realize writing a book will never pay me the money I get from being a Top Trainer. However, after looking at the garbage these so-called "Star Trainers" put on the market, I thought it was time to write something that's not full of quick tricks, basic workouts, fancy fluff or shiny gadgets. The Fitness and Food Actions in this book are written from my 24 years of knowledge (college and life) and experiences (fitness trainer and competitive wrestler). Since 21 years old, I've not only trained Pro and Olympic Athletes, but I have been personally coached by some of the world's best trainers from all over the world as a wrestler. No matter if it's been boxing, wrestling, strength training or any other exercise modality. I always searched for the best training. Now, I've decided to give you some of what I've learned that has helped hundreds of guys, just like you, get in the best shape of their life.

Fuck doing tricep dips on a chair, lifting your leg up like a dog pissing on a hydrant, eating protein bars full of shit and screw acting like your 18 with your arms out to your side. This book is for guys who are 30 plus years old who don't have to follow the though process that your days of being fit are over. I'm 45 and still wrestle division 1A college wrestlers, spar professional boxers, run 6-8 miles a day and masturbate at least twice a week, lol.

The only way this will fail for you is if — and only if — you don't <u>put at least **one** of these snippets</u> into action. I don't care if you're fat, skinny, weak, unfit, fit or anything in between. There is at least one piece of information you can use in this book to feel and look better!

PLEASE NOTE: I realize losing weight and/or getting into shape is not just about eating right and exercising. There are many factors (physical, psychological, time, money, etc.) that can hinder you from reaching your goal. Do not take any of my comments to heart, as they are meant to motivate you (in a weird way with no sugar coating). I really do have a passion for helping anyone who wants to reach their fitness and dietary goal (s). I hope I can help you with this book. Please don't cry.

WANT TO GET INTO THE BEST SHAPE OF YOUR LIFE- FAST?
BOOK A CALL CLICK HERE

How To Use This Book:

Read this book a few times. Highlight the actions that pertain to you and your goals. Bring this book with you to the gym or your workout room. I recommend buying the printed version. The workout plans will give you amazing results. A printed version will allow you to take notes and mark up as needed.

DOUGS' DISCLAIMER:

"If you're just into reading fitness books with a lot of feel good shit. Fit Actions is not for you! So, Take Fucking Action. Don't Cry. Man up and get results! "

-Doug Bennett

THE MEDICAL DISCLAIMER:

I'm not a doctor nor do I pretend to be. Always consult with your primary health care professional before starting any diet or fitness program. The material in this book, **Fit Actions** written by Doug Bennett, is for informational purposes only. Use any of the information (diet, exercise and techniques) in this book at your own risk. Each individual needs vary from person to person. The information in this book is not a personal diet or exercise plan. The author, Doug Bennett, expressly disclaims responsibility for any injury or adverse effects that may be caused from the use or application of information in this book. Always stop exercising immediately and call for medical help if you feel dizzy, weak or faint.

Ok, now that we got that out of the way, onward.

GET READY
TO GET
READY !

1

GET READY ACTION NO. 1

SET YOUR GOALS

Goal setting has been studied and written about for decades. You probably know more about goal setting theory than I do. However, the majority of people set their goal(s) too high or simply don't take action. The good old sayings "All talk and no action!" or "Analysis Paralysis" apply over and over.

Below is what works for me.

"Shut Up and Do it!"

- Set weekly goals at four-week increments. Don't do too many things at once.
- Set a main goal and then break it up in steps (specific actions) to outline how you're going to achieve that goal.
- Always have a Plan B (excuse plan) in case something comes up that will disrupt that goal. This will help you determine the action needed to stay on goal.

Workout Goal Setting:

Example 4-week goal setting for a beginner:

Beginners:

WEEK 1-2

Broad Goal: I'm going to train 2 days per week for the next 2 weeks at the gym!

Specific: I'm going to train every Monday (5:30 a.m.) before work and Thursday (6:00 p.m.) after work.

Specific A: I'm going to train my whole body both days for 30 minutes total by focusing on 20 minutes of cardio (walking, jogging, jumping jacks) and 10 minutes of body exercises (push-ups, sit-ups, crunches, etc.)

WEEK 3-4

Broad Goal: I'm going to add a day (Saturday) to my weekly training that includes all weights for 30 minutes at my gym.

Specific: I'm going to focus on my chest, shoulders and arms on this day.

Specific A: I'm going to do 8 sets for my chest, 3 sets for my shoulders, 6 sets for my biceps, and 3 sets for my triceps.

Excuse Plan: If something comes up, I'm going to train the very next day instead.

HABIT: Write out a plan every month for the next six months.

SHORTCUT: Download a goal-setting app that keeps you accountable.

Tip: Goal setting is important. Give yourself a reward for each goal you accomplish and a penalty for each one not met. Example Reward: Get a deep tissue massage if you meet all month 1 goals. Example Penalty: Run an extra mile and/or do 100 extra push-ups if you do not meet your goals.

Action Plan:

1. Print out your goal and sign it.
2. Write out your program and print it.
3. File it and send a copy to your email. Download it to your phone and save it as a pic. This way you can never use the excuse you forgot it.

If you need coddling, show your goal to someone who will keep you accountable.

2

GET READY ACTION NO. 2

BUY A HEART RATE MONITOR

First, make sure you get a clearance from your doctor to participate in any cardiovascular activity that will increase your heart rate above normal daily activity.

A heart rate monitor is a cheap and effective fitness tool to keep you motivated and accountable to your fitness goals. You'll rarely ever see a professional cyclist, runner or triathlete without a heart rate monitor. All for a good reason. You can scientifically improve your speed, endurance and capacity to withstand strenuous fitness levels.

Twenty-five years ago while in college, my exercise science classes taught that to get a quick approximate max heart rate, you could simply take age and subtract if from 220. Example: A 40-year-old man would have a max heart rate of approximately 180.

In reality, a max heart rate is individual specific based on fitness level, sport, medical history, etc.

I believe the best reason to wear a heart rate monitor is to get a real indication of how hard you're working based on a true number rather than a psychological cue saying, "I'm at my limit. I'm too tired to go harder!" The reality is that you may be able to go a little harder or longer.

So, with that said…

How Do You Calculate Your Maximum Heart Rate (if and only if you have no cardiac risk factors)?

Here Are Two Suggestions:

1. Hire a running coach and have him time you on a track.
2. Yourself: Sprint 100 yards with your heart rate monitor and take a reading immediately after the end mark. You should be out of breath. If not, walk back to the 50-yard line and sprint back to the end line.

Uses for Your Heart Rate Monitor:

1. Running:

*Beginners: Jog until you reach 75 % your max heart rate and then walk/trot until your heart rate is at 60-65% for few minutes. Pick up the pace back to 75% until it starts to elevate. Rinse and repeat for 1-3 miles based upon your individual fitness level. Every week increase the frequency of the days you run and the time you keep your heart rate up to 70% of max.

Summary: Keep heart rate 60-75% max heart rate.

*Intermediate to Advanced: This is where you can really improve your times by using your heart rate monitor to guide you between easy running days, long distance days, and short, intense running sessions.

Easy days running with tempos (5 minutes 60%, 1 minute 80%, 30 seconds 95% and repeat).

Longer days running at 65-75% of max.

Short, Intense days running at 85-95% of max.

*These are all just examples. If you are serious about being a runner, it's worth hiring a running coach who is well educated for your individual running goals to prevent injury. They can help you pick the right running shoe, proper running tempos and much more...

2. Weight Loss:

It's best to vary your heart rate to lose weight. Yes, keeping your heart rate at 75%-85% (aerobic zone) is important, but it's also important to increase the duration of your workouts if possible. Obviously, if you're time limited, keep your heart rate high. The more intense the workout, the more your body has to work and the more calories you'll burn. Oh yeah, calories do matter if your body is storing them rather than using them for bodily function (a.k.a. building muscle). If you think varying days between HIIT type of workouts and other days of long runs won't help. You're wrong! This is just for trainers who want to make themselves feel good because they do mountain climbers all day. They obviously have never wrestled or done a contact sport. They just want to look pretty and tough.

Example:

Leg Circuit to Burn Calories

Always warm up with a light jog, stretching (back, knees, legs, etc.).

(Perform the 4 exercises below as shown, no rest. Then rest 1 minute and repeat program again 2-3x)

1. Heavy Squat (5 reps at 90% max weight*).
2. Speed Rope 3 minutes (every 30 seconds bring your heart rate up to 85% for 30 seconds)
3. Moderate Squat (15 reps at 70% max weight)
4. Mountain Climbers 1 minute (last 30 seconds bring your heart rate up to 85%)

*Max weight = best form for 1 repetition.

HABIT: Use the heart rate monitor every time you do cardio to show progression and keep in the most effective range required of your goal. Effective use of a heart rate monitor is a great way to shed pounds.

TIP: I recommend buying a basic heart rate monitor. No need to get fancy unless you're a high-level athlete. A Garmin Heart Rate Monitor will cover all your needs.

SHORTCUT: If you don't want to buy a heart rate monitor, perform a full sprint on a track or field and sprint until it would be difficult to hold a conversation. Immediately take your radial pulse (on the inside of the wrist) with your two fingers (never your thumb). Press lightly on the wrist at the base of your thumb. You should feel the pulse right away. Count it for sixty seconds. This heart rate reading should be close to your max heart rate.

Want results like Andrew?

90 Days lost 47 lbs., 6 months transformed his body from 46 % Body Fat to 19%, Couldn't do a push up and now bangs out 4 x 50 at 52 Years Old.

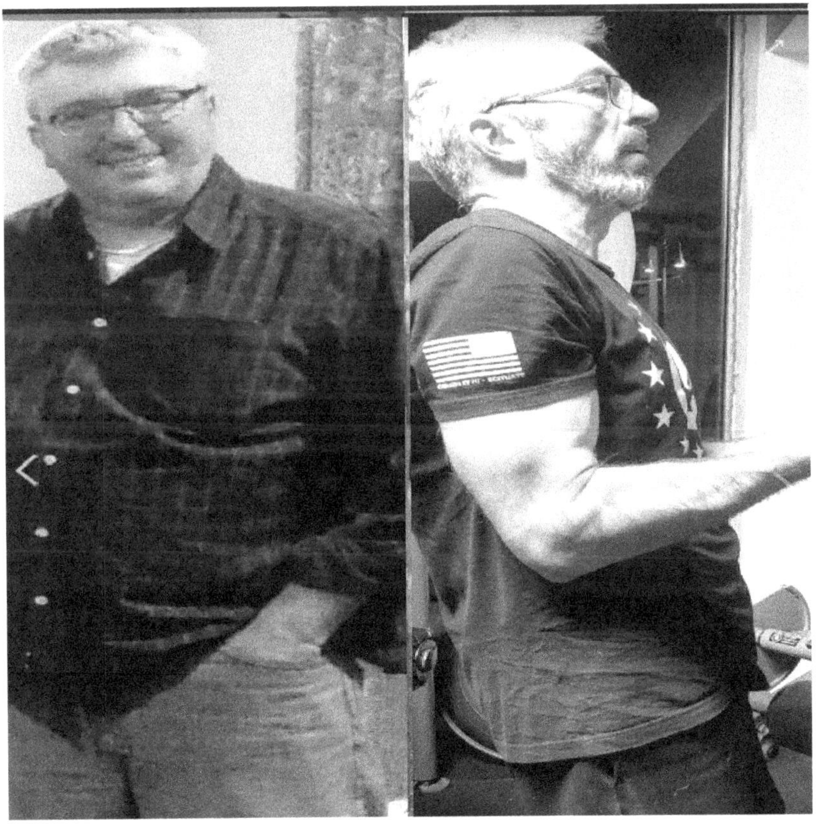

COACHEDFITRX.COM

3

GET READY ACTION NO. 3

GET THE RIGHT GEAR

Yes, I know. This is so elementary, but many people don't get the right gear. Hence, it stops them from getting their workout in or it becomes an excuse. It's not bad weather. It's bad workout gear.

Wearing the proper gear is crucial when it comes to training outside, especially in the winter. Don't let the weather affect your motivation and workouts. Make sure you get the right gear that will protect you from the cold, rain, wind, etc. Oh yeah, don't forget about reflective gear if you're getting home late. Outside training really is the best way to train hard core (running, biking, swimming, etc.).

Hence, you should have the right gear for both the summer and winter if you're going to train outside. In the winter, you'll warm up at least 15 degrees if you're training hard, so dress accordingly. In the summer, you need to stay cool and have gear that doesn't absorb the sweat.

Growing up I would have said, "You're a pussy if you have to wear that special shirt. Who cares what you look like?" Well, years have passed and I now get it. I eat my words and now know from experience that wearing the right clothes makes a difference.

Now, don't get me wrong. It won't help you win a title. However, it can make small changes in your performance. Example: if you run with too many layers, you can affect your rhythm. If you wear a shirt that's too tight when boxing or playing basketball, you can inhibit free motion of your shoulder and arm, which in turn will cause you to underperform.

HABIT: Wear clothes that allow you to perform at your best level while still looking good. Wearing the right clothes can also help you get mentally prepared to train hard and get down to business.

TIP: Buy your workout gear at discount stores like Marshalls, T.J. Maxx, Old Navy or your favorite online store when there are close outs (REI, Eastern Mountain Sports, Amazon, etc.) to sell off last year's gear. If you have to pay top dollar to get workout pants that fit just right, do it. Quality will last for many years. I always buy at the end of the season for next season. Example: I recently bought all my gear for the next winter season two weeks after Christmas. I saved money and got the top gear cheaply.

SHORTCUT: Buy one and even two of each.

Buy 1:

- Tank tops
- Short sleeve shirts
- Long sleeve shirts
- Cross Training Shoes
- Wind breaker

- Fleece Pull Over
- Rain Coat
- Running hat
- Running gloves

Buy 2 if possible:

- Workout pants (light and lined for winter)
- Training shorts
- Under gear (long and short)
- Running shorts and pants
- Workout socks (high and short)
- Running Shoes (if you're serious about running, it's best to have two pairs in case one gets wet. Wet running shoes can lose their support.)

GET HELP HERE >> COACHEDFITRX.COM

4

GET READY ACTION NO. 4

BUILD A HOME GYM

You don't need much equipment or space to get fit at home. Keep some equipment at home even if you have a gym membership. I personally have a heavy bag, dumbbells, wrestling mats, pull-up bar, jump rope, medicine balls, fitness ball and a double end bag in my basement.

Find a comfortable and safe area where you can train. Try to choose an area that you can use at any time of the day. It's of no use if you can't wake up and work out without waking everyone else up.

Minimum Equipment Needed:

- 2-3 dumbbell sets. (light, moderate, heavy)
- Jump rope
- Medicine ball
- Fitness Ball
- Pull-Up Bar

Optimum Add On:

- Treadmill
- Bosu
- Heavy Bag
- Power Rack and/or Smith Machine
- Decline Sit-Up Bench
- Weight rack and Dumbbells (5 to 60 lbs.)
- Adjustable Bench and/or bench with rack.
- Dip n Pull-Up station

HABIT: Perform pull-ups, jumping rope and push-ups every day at home. Best if you can do morning and night (10-15 minutes each). Example: perform 1-5 pull-ups then drop down and do 5-25 push-ups and repeat for 3-5 minutes. Follow-up with 5-10 minutes of jumping rope.

TIP: Don't buy a universal gym unless you have lots of room and money to burn. Keep to the basics.

SHORTCUT: Best bang for your buck — heavy bag, jump rope, boxing gloves and pull-up bar. Just thirty minutes of 3-5 rounds of mixing it up will help you drop weight fast and keep your attention.

5

GET READY ACTION NO. 5

GET A GYM MEMBERSHIP

If you want to really look like a body builder, you have to train like one and get a membership to a club with lots of weights, space and machines. A home gym and a gym membership are key to changing it up. I personally use my home gym and the outside trails, hills, local school stairs, etc.

HABIT: Use your membership at least three times per week for all your heavy lifts.

TIP: Sign up to a $10.00 - $20.00 membership/month gym with no frills, just good old weights and cardio equipment.

SHORTCUT: Join during the best months to get the best deals. Gyms love to give deals during their lull times like the summer. Obviously, $ 10.00/month is no big deal. Especially if you miss a month or two due to work, family, etc.

FITNESS ACTIONS

READY! SET! TAKE ACTION!

"Just reading these tips and not taking action (not performing the workouts, etc.) will not do shit. Reading why we get fat, blah, blah is for the mind, this book is to get your ass into shape, period. "

-Doug Bennett

1

FITNESS ACTION NO. 1

WARM UP

Warming up is very important. Most people are eager to get right after it. I don't blame you. Yet as you get older, you learn that warming up before doing any strenuous exercise is key to preventing injury. I remember as a kid and in college showing up for wrestling practice late. I would throw on my shoes and grapple. Never an injury and always ready for battle. Yet, after twenty-eight I noticed this didn't work anymore. I started to get nagging tendon and ligament issues that would have never happened before. How many friends do you know who have jumped up for a ball or started to run and tore their Achilles? Probably, at least one.

What to Do about It:

You should warm up before exercising and getting a sweat going. I believe warming up is more important than stretching. Below are some warm ups to do before some common training exercises.

Action Plan:

Boxing: jump rope, double end bag, hitting mitts, shadow boxing, jogging.

Sprinting: jogging, high knee running, jumping jacks, 50% max runs.

Tennis: jogging, side shuffles, jumping jacks, racquet swings.

Weight Training: jump rope, treadmill walking or jogging on incline, push-ups, bike and elliptical

Golf: Swinging, toe touches

Basketball: jump rope, jogging, layups, bounding leaps

Boot Camp: jogging, push-ups, jump rope, jumping jacks

HABIT: Perform ten minutes of warm up before any exercise.

TIP: One minute of jumping jacks in the morning is a great to start the day.

SHORTCUT: Ten jumping jacks, ten high knee runs and ten low squats. Repeat 10x.

BOTTOM-LINE: **Get sweating.**

COACHEDFITRX.COM

2

FITNESS ACTION NO. 2

HYDRATE

Water is vital for muscle development, metabolic processes and overall health. Your muscles are comprised of approximately 70-75% water. Below is why you should drink water:

- **Distributes nutrients.** Water helps transport nutrients and enzymes needed for muscle development (protein synthesis). **You can increase gains from a heavy lifting day by simply taking in adequate water to transport the amino acids (a.k.a. lean protein building blocks) you'll eat that day. RIGHT!**

- **Keeps you energized.** Dehydration can cause you to feel sluggish and lethargic. **Your workouts will suck!** Remember, blood transports oxygen. Blood is made up of 83% water.

- **Aids in keeping you lubricated (not talking sexually).** Physically helps your joints by making up synovial fluid, which keeps your joints lubricated (not stiff). Thus, helping to prevent injury.

- **Increases your sperm count to make the babies.** Yes, it MAY help increase your sperm count.

- **Helps prevent injuries from supplements**. Helps prevent injury when taking supplements and eating foods that zap water from your muscles. Caffeine, Creatine Monohydrate and Nitric Oxide can all decrease the water content in your muscles, which can lead to cramping, muscle strains and even tears.
- **Critical for fat burning**. If your body is dehydrated, your liver (the major fat burning organ that removes fatty acids from the blood stream and regulates both fat and carbohydrate metabolism) will become distressed. **This leads to a slowdown of the fat burning process**.

What to Do about It:

- Don't count on other liquids as your water source. Smoothies, Coffee, Carbonated Water, etc. all have water, but don't put them into the equation. Drink pure spring water if possible.
- Purchase a case of spring water and store it in an accessible place — work, car trunk, kitchen, etc.
- Never keep water stored in a plastic container in direct sunlight.
- If you're training like a beast, you can even walk around the gym with a gallon of it. You may look like a meathead, but you'll be hydrated.
- If you're in a yuppie gym, walk around with a water bottle and knock guys out with it every time they look down on you.
- Keep a case of coconut water (unsweetened) in your house to grab one each day. Coconut water contains lots of good natural electrolytes and minerals. Make sure it's from a good source as not all coconut water is the same.

HABIT: You're a workout guy. So, drink more than the typically recommended amount of water for the average guy — eight eight-ounce glasses of water a day.

Start every morning with a tall glass of room temperature water, preferably with a squeeze of fresh lemon juice.

Drink at least 10 ounces of pure water every two hours. Aim for a minimum of ten eight-ounce glasses of water a day.

TIP: Drink water throughout your workout. Drink an electrolyte beverage like coconut water during any strenuous long distance training session to avoid electrolyte imbalances caused by sweating and just drinking pure water.

SHORTCUT: Daily

Drink 1-10 ounce glass of water with an Emergen-C supplement that contains 1,000 mg Vitamin C and electrolytes.

Drink 1-10 ounce glass of water with fresh lemon juice.

Drink 6 to 8 – 10 ounce glasses of just pure room temperature water.

BOTTOM-LINE: Force yourself to drink water. It improves muscle health and increases your metabolism! If you don't like the taste now, you'll love it if you drink it every day for a week or two.

COACHEDFITRX.COM

3

FITNESS ACTION NO. 3

STRETCHING

This goes hand and hand with warming up. It's best to warm up and then lightly stretch. Does this mean you have to perform two hours of yoga every day? Hell no. Although, I'd be envious if you have two hours to devote to yoga. In a busy life, warming up and then stretching for five to ten minutes before training should suffice. Stretching is the key to life, especially after thirty. The aging process is brutal, and you'll notice that your younger years of splits and placing your foot behind your head just isn't happening anymore (ha-ha).

Anyhow, stretching is critical. Here's a lifelong lesson from me.

I started training with heavy weights at twelve years old in my basement. At fourteen, I pushed more weight than my tendons and muscles could probably handle. Then came wrestling. So, my tightly bound muscles were now being pulled and pushed to a whole new level, which caused microscopic tears at the cellular level.

Four more years of heavy weight training, wrestling and no stretching = Myofascitis (inflammation of the muscle cells).

In college, when my muscles got inflamed from a lack of sleep and an intense wrestling session, the pain was so excruciating I could barely lift my arms to drive my car. I could press 325 lbs. when I weighed 140 lbs., and if my muscles got inflamed I could barely do a push-up.

Learn from my mistake. Find time to stretch, especially if you plan to train aggressively.

HABIT: Stretch after a warm shower every day for 3-5 minutes. Optimum 10 minutes.

TIP: Warm up and stretch throughout your exercise. Emphasize stretching the body part you're working on that day. Example of training legs stretch: Hamstrings — place your foot high up so that it's higher than thigh level with locked knee, and flexed toe. Quads — stand and pull laces up toward butt and hold stretch 30 sec. – 1 min.

Stretch Muscles for Each Below:

- Hamstring
- Calves
- Biceps
- Triceps
- Quads
- Lower Back
- Upper Back

SHORTCUT: Take a yoga or martial arts class 2-3x week to increase flexibility. Note: online yoga classes and apps are available too.

BOTTOM-LINE: Stretch in the morning and night.

4

FITNESS ACTION NO. 4

PERFORM CARDIO FOR WEIGHT LOSS PERFORM MINIMAL CARDIO FOR WEIGHT GAIN

Weight Loss

First, let's get something straight. You can build muscle and lose some weight without performing long cardio sessions.

However, please, don't listen to the crap that you can get ripped by **_working out only 30 minutes per week_** while never doing cardio and eating all the bacon you want.

Yes, if you eat fewer carbs, you'll lose some water weight and fat, but you'll still be a slow, lazy, fat ass slob who won't last 30 seconds in a fight or even run a minute without holding your chest.

Cardio isn't just about losing weight. It makes you feel better and certainly makes you healthier.

I don't care if you just walk in place and suck your thumb. It's simple. **Move your ass.**

So, with that off my chest…let's go on.

Weight Gain

If you want to gain weight (a.k.a Big Muscles), you should lift heavy, eat a lot of calories (good calories, 60% protein broken up into small meals), take some supplements and train like an animal. Not rocket science but it takes a lot of discipline, hard work and the right workout. Oh yeah, a little genetics helps too.

I'll discuss weight gain later.

Cardio Session Samples

Below are some simple samples on how to **mix it up** to drop some pounds and tighten up whether you're working out outside, at home, on travel and/or at the gym.

OUTSIDE CARDIO WORKOUTS

Mix Short Duration intense days with *longer cardio days, if applicable, for best results.

*Longer Cardio Days for you may simply involve jogging and walking for 45 minutes. That's ok. This is about you.

Short Day Cardio:

- Jump Rope 3 x 3 min. with 1 min rest between sets. Every 30 seconds speed up your jumping for 15 seconds.

- Jog 1 mile
- *Sprints 6 x 25 yards, 4 x 50 yards, 8 x 100 yards, rest 30 seconds to 1 minute between sprints
- Jog 1 to 3 miles

***Please read Fitness Action #14-**Sprinting before you integrate sprinting into your workout plan.

Long Day Cardio:

Jog 3-8 miles. Every quarter of a mile, sprint for 30 seconds at 80% (80% effort of a full sprint). Find a running route that includes hills.

Obviously, everyone's fitness level is different. Some of you may power walk and some of you may jog 12 miles plus for your longer days.

Simply mix the shit up (cardio) and get after it!

Home or Hotel Cardio Workouts (No Equipment Needed):

Fitness Level:	Beginner	Fit Guy
	Repeat 3x	Repeat 5x

Fitness Training 1

1. Jump rope or Jacks	1 min	3 min
2. Mountain Climbers	1 min	1 min
3. Running High Knees	2 min	1 min
4. Speed Jump Rope	30 seconds	1 min
5. High Speed *Straight Punches	30 seconds	1 min, hold 2lbs
6. Push ups	10 to 25	25 to 50

NO GYM WORKOUTS

Fitness Training 2

	Beginner repeat 2x	Fit Guy repeat 3 to 5 x
1. Jump rope or Jacks	1 min	3 min
2. Burpees w/ push-up	1 min	1 min
3. Running High Knees	1 min	3 min
4. Mountain Climbers	30 seconds	1 min
5. Burpees w high knees (10)	Skip	1 min
6. Skating	1 min	1 min
7. Jumping Squat plus push ups	10 plus 2	10 plus 10

repeat squat plus push ups for beginner and advanced 10 x

Fitness Training 3

	Beginner	Fit Guy
1. Jump Rope	2 min	3 min
2. Shadow Box	2 min	3 min
3. Burpee w/ 4 punches	1 min	1 min
4. Speed Jump Rope	30 sec.	1 min
5. Leap Frog	1 min	2 min

Have extra time to work out after each one of these training sessions?

Simply, power walk or jog 2 or more miles (time and fitness level dependent).

Gym or Home Cardio Workouts (Equipment)

Fitness Training 1 (Short)

Warm Up:

Treadmill (no incline)	4 min trot	4 min jog
Treadmill *(incline 2-5)	1 min power walk/trot	1 min jog
	Repeat #1 to # 6, 3 x	**Repeat #1 to #6, 3x**
1. Treadmill (no incline)	1 min walk	1 min walk
2. Treadmill *(incline 6-10)	1 min power walk/trot	2 min jog (speed 4.0 – 5.0)

*(Incline Running) Hold on to the cross bar the entire time and <u>concentrate on pushing off feet hard</u> as if you're driving the belt behind you. Keep the treadmill speed slow so you can concentrate on pushing the belt back.

3. Jump Rope	1 minute	3 minutes
4. Bike Standing	1 minute	*3 minutes

*vary the bike tension every 30 seconds between low tension to high tension (3 to 8) on scale of 1 to 10, 1 being easiest and 10 being most difficult to spin.

| 5. Speed Jump Rope | 1 minute | 1 minute |

Repeat all exercises #1 to #6, 2 more times

Fitness Training 2 (Long)

1. Treadmill	3 min power walk	3 min trot
	10 min walk/trot	15 min jog
2. Incline 3	15 min walk/trot	Skip
3. Incline 5	Skip	10 min jog
4. Incline 2	Skip	15 min jog
5. Incline 1	Skip	1-3 min sprint @ 70% max
		2-5 min sprint @80% max
6. Jump Rope	1-2 min	6 min
7. *Lateral X Overs Bosu	Skip	3 min
8. Rest 1 min	rest	rest
9. Lateral X Overs Bosu	1 Minute	3 min
10. Bike or Rowing Machine	Skip	3-5 minutes

*Lateral X-Overs Bosu: Place one foot on the ground and one foot on the top of a Bosu (half globe exercise apparatus, google it). Push off the Bosu with your foot on the top and replace this foot with the foot on the ground. Repeat this activity and go back and forth in a lateral manner. Make sure you push yourself up high with the foot on the Bosu. Keep weight on that foot. Don't stay on the balls of your feet. You can do this with a block or bench also If you don't have a Bosu.

HABIT: Commit to minimum 30 minutes of <u>daily cardio</u> for the next 120 days.

TIP:

- Buy a piece of equipment that you'll use every day to stay committed to cardio.
- Before purchasing expensive cardio equipment (treadmills, elliptical, rowing machines):
    - Search Craig's List for used equipment.
    - Call local gyms, hotels, personal training studios, etc. to see if they are getting rid of used cardio Machines.
- Keep a jump rope, running shoes and workout clothes in a duffel bag at all times (car, travel, etc.
- No excuses.

SHORTCUTS: All are based upon your individual goal.

Lose Weight: One or a combination of Power Walking/Running/Sprinting/Plyometrics for minimum of 30-40 minutes per day/5-6 days per week. Best formula: add 2 days of HIIT (High Intensity Interval

Training, see #16 along with longer cardio days).

Gain Weight: Walking/Biking/Jump Rope for maximum 15-20 minutes per day/3 days per week.

Gain Strength: Walking/Light Jog/Jump Rope for maximum 15 minutes per day after your workout, preferably on off days of heavy/major lifts (dead lifts, cleans, bench, etc.).

Warm up with 5 to 10 minutes light cardio.

Get Ripped: Sprinting/Jogging/Jump Rope for 20-30 minutes per day/3-5 days per week.

Best formula: add 1-2 days of HIIT (High Intensity Interval Training, see #16) and tempo training. **NOTE:** You should be lifting heavy at least 2 days per week with major lifts (bench, squat, dead lifts, etc.).

Build Endurance: One or a combination of Jogging/Sprinting/Hill Sprinting/Jump Rope/Biking/Rowing/Swimming combining short distance and long distance training days. Dependent on your goal and fitness level (i.e., triathlon, marathon, etc.).

BOTTOM-LINE: **Move it.**

COACHEDFITRX.COM

5

FITNESS ACTION NO. 5

LEARN TO BOX THE RIGHT WAY

Do me a favor. Please don't attend a boxing boot camp or some other girly boxing class and call yourself a boxer. Yes, it's fun to hit stuff. Just remember, boxing really isn't one of the sports where you just win or lose. If you lose, you probably got rocked or knocked out. Your best bet is to hire a real boxing coach for 5 -10 sessions to learn the basics. For those who just want to get fit, boxing is a great way to work out no matter where you go (travel, home, gym). If you learn the right way, you can still get a great workout without heavy bags, speed bags or even gloves. Shadow boxing is the best way to work on technique while burning calories.

HABIT: Shadow box for five three-minute rounds every day. Work on technique and get a sweat going.

TIP: Learn footwork first. Then learn how to throw your punches with your body, not just your arms. Improve your speed once you get the technique down. Speed is power.

<u>Mix up your rounds with:</u>

1. **Heavy bag** – move with it and don't stand in front of it like 99% of the dopes who teach boxing. Mix up rounds with power punches and speed combinations.
2. **Double end bag** – best training apparatus for accuracy, speed and movement. Again, don't just stand in front of it.
3. **Jump Rope** – (see fitness action #16)
4. **Foot Work and movement** – lateral movement plus front to back while always keeping a good stance. Never crossing feet.
5. **Ab Work** – decline sit-ups, leg raises, hanging leg raises, sit-ups with punching, medicine ball throws (see fitness action #24)
6. **Speed Bag** – Work on technique before speed. Tap at all angles and work on keeping arms up to train shoulder endurance. Great for hand and eye coordination.

SHORTCUT: Find a boxing gym in your area that has real boxing coaches and trainers. Not your local trainer who holds up mitts and says, "I box!" **FUCK HIM.** I'm sick of imposters.

Yet, if you want to use boxing to complement weight training, you can use the schedule below.

Box for 20-30 minutes every other day combined with running/power walking/sprinting, etc. in between 2-3 days of heavy weights.

EXAMPLE:

Day 1: Heavy/Low Rep Upper Body

Day 2: Boxing/Cardio

Day 3: Heavy Lower/Low Rep Body

Day 4: Boxing/Cardio

Day 5: Moderate/High Rep Upper n Lower Body

Day 6: Long Endurance Cardio Session

Day 7: Rest or Yoga

BOTTOM-LINE: Everyone should learn how to defend themselves and throw a punch. Plus, you'll get in great shape.

6

FITNESS ACTION NO. 6

MIX UP CARDIO TO TRAIN BODY PARTS

Bring up your heart rate! This is why I suggest purchasing a heart rate monitor if you're serious about upping your game. Keeping your heart rate at 60-80% your max heart rate is key to burning fat during a longer cardio session (45 minutes plus...). Increasing your heart rate at 70-90% for a short burst of 1 to 30 minutes (dependent on medical clearance from your primary physician) is great to both increase your cardiac endurance, VO_2 max and to burn calories.

Below are some great ways to increase your metabolic endurance for both your heart and body parts:

Build Legs:

Sprinting, *Plyometrics, Trail Running, Kicking, Hills and Stairs, Biking, Ladder

Build Arms and Shoulders:

Boxing, Boot Camp Exercises (mountain climbers, burpees, bear crawl), Swimming

Build Abs:

Boxing, Boot Camp Exercises (mountain climbers, burpees, bear crawl), Sprinting, *Plyometrics

*Plyometrics: box jumps, leapfrogs, hops, vertical Jumping, Burpee with a jump

HABIT: Perform daily: 5 - 10 burpees, at least 50 mountain climbers, at least 10 vertical Jumps, and straight punches with 2 lb. weights 1 min (use your body).

TIP: Best to be done later in the day when warmed up. Never perform any jumping activity without warming up your calves, knees, lower back and Achilles tendon.

SHORTCUT: Join an outside boot camp class once a week.

BOTTOM LINE: **Build up your endurance** by mixing up your cardio.

7

FITNESS ACTION NO. 7

LIFT HEAVY

I believe lifting heavy is similar to sprinting. Give it all you got! Fuck lifting light weights for 50 reps to build muscle. The only reason to do reps of 25 and greater is if you're in your third phase of getting ready for a fight, rehabbing an injury or in a triathlete training program.

There Are So Many Benefits from Lifting Heavy:

1. Cuts workout time.
2. Creates rock hard, dense, muscles.
3. Weight Gain
4. Spikes testosterone for bigger muscle and hard-ons.
5. Increase Strength
6. Lowers Body Fat

Here Are Some Key Ideas to Know:

1. Lifting at 70% to 90% of your max is a great way to build muscle and strength.

2. Lifting heavy is one thing. However, the reps you perform are all goal dependent.

3. For strength: 1-3 reps / 4-6 sets with 3-5 minutes rest between sets.

4. Mass and Strength: 4-8 reps / 5-6 sets with 2-3 minutes rest between sets.

5. Endurance: 1 to 3 sets – perform 3-5 reps with 2-4 minutes rest between sets. Sets 4 and 5 – perform 3-5 reps followed by the same exercise or a secondary exercise with less weight (drop set) and perform good form reps to failure. Example: One Arm Row for sets 4 and 5. Perform 5 reps at 100 lbs. (90% max) and immediately follow with 70 pounds until failure or immediately follow the one arm row 5 reps with chin-ups (palms facing you) until failure.

6. Always perform a warm-up set before lifting heavy and stretch the muscles you're training.

7. Goal Dependent.

8. Rest 2-5 minutes between sets by doing crunches, stretching and/or another ab exercise.

NOTE:

Best to keep reps between 4-6 reps. If you can only do 2 reps @ 90% max, drop down to 80% max and get the last 3 to 4 reps.

Example:

Flat Bench: **Set1:** 225 **Set 2:** 235 **Set 3:**235 **Set 4: 235** followed by push-ups until failure.

Set 5: 225 followed by dips until failure.

9. You should be able to do every rep with good to great form.

10. Always lift with a spotter (training partner who can lift the weight if needed).

11. Rest 2-3 days between Heavy Days for similar body parts. The heavier you lift, the longer you should wait. Also, if you're just beginning to lift heavy, keep your sets between 2 to 3 and train one body part heavy once per week for a month or even two before proceeding to 2x per week per body part.

12. Lift heavy with basic exercises only. **See Below for exercises of 3-5 reps**.

EXERCISES FOR EACH BODY PART TO LIFT HEAVY FOR STRENGTH AND MUSCLE

Legs: Squat, Back Leg Curls, Leg Press, *Cleans, *Deadlifts

Chest: Flat Press, Incline Press, Flat Dumbbell Press, Incline Dumbbell Press, *Weighted Dips

Back: Low Rows, *Deadlifts, *Cleans, One Arm Rows, *Weighted Pull-Ups

Shoulders: Straight Bar Press, *Clean and Press, Sitting Dumbbell Press

Neck: *Upright rows, Shrugs

Calves: *Standing press

Triceps: *Close Grip Press with bar

* Advanced only. Never perform these without a spotter, perfect form or at least a good foundation of muscle development. Serious injury can result without the proper form, instruction and program.

HABIT: Lift Heavy once per week if you're beginner, twice per week if you're an advanced lifter.

TIP: Try doing drop sets one workout a week. Lift 95% for one rep, drop to 80-90% for 5-8 reps.

Most all of my muscle that I've kept from my younger years of training is from lifting heavy. I personally try to lift heavy twice per week and lighter once per week. The max I lift is 30 minutes per workout. I like to keep strength and agility to box and wrestle.

SHORTCUT: If you're a beginner, make sure you don't perform your one rep max without at least a month of training. Also, warm up before trying your 1 rep max to prevent tendon, ligament and muscle injury. To increase your strength, have a friend help you by doing this:

Perform 2-3 reps on your own with 90% max. For the last 2-3 reps, have your friend help you up so it's now approximately 50% max. However, you now will perform a negative rep (opposite of the action to perform the rep) going down as slowly as possible. Once you are at the beginning of a new rep again your friend will help you get it back up and repeat.

Example:

Bench press

Perform 2-3 reps at 225 pressing up with acceleration and decelerating the bar down to the chest for 2-3 seconds. Now, at rep 3 your friend will slightly help you get the bar up but now you'll fight the lowering of the bar down to your chest. So it will take now 5-6 seconds to hit your chest. Once it hits your chest, you'll press with all your might, but your friend will help assist it up and you'll repeat for the next 2-3 reps. Make sure your friend is strong enough to assist in this type of training.

BOTTOM-LINE: **Add heavy days to your workouts.**

FITNESS REALITY CHECK:

IF YOU LOST YOUR LEGS TODAY. WHAT WOULD YOU DO TOMORROW, IF I GAVE THEM BACK TO YOU?
YOU'D PROBABLY RUN LIKE YOU NEVER HAVE BEFORE. START USING YOUR LEGS. TAKE ACTION NOW.

8

FITNESS ACTION NO. 8

HOLD THE MOMENT

One sure way to increase your gains while lifting is to hold the exercise rep at the end of the movement for 2 to 4 seconds and squeeze the muscle you're training. This brings more blood into the area and creates a muscle fiber activation that leads to better results.

I cringe when I see people at the gym throw weights up and down with no form. Shaping your muscles takes good form. It's ok to blast the weight up, but make sure you hold it for 2-3 seconds and then let it down at a slower pace. Hold the moment is not to be performed with a heavy set. Good form is always important (Explode up/down, hold and lower/release slower).

Below is a Sample of Exercises to do on Your Muscle Building Day:

Chest:

Bar Bell, Hammer Strength (unilateral press) and/or Dumbbells Press: Start at Top Position. Let down slowly. Reach the bottom and blast up. Hold at top and squeeze your pecs 2-3 seconds. You can do two things on top: keep a slight bend in elbow and squeeze or lock out your elbow to get a full contraction (I recommend). Just don't straighten out so fat that you overextend your reach which makes your shoulder blades rotate to forward. Squeezing a contraction of your chest works best on top with a heavy weight (spotter will help you do heavier weights).

Cable, Pec Deck and/or Dumbbell Flies: Change it up. Start heavy and drop down to a lighter weight. Do 5 to 6 reps heavy and 10 to 15 reps lighter (you should be struggling on your last rep). When you squeeze your pecs on the end of the adduction movement (bringing cables or dumbbells towards each other) Keep the handles of the cable machine or pec deck handles or pads 1 inch away from each other to keep constant tension on pecs (don't let them touch, unless you want to do a pulse movement for the last few reps. Once you have the handles 1 inch away from each other, hold them there and squeeze your chest for 2-3 seconds. Then slowly release the handles until you feel a good stretch in your chest, then hold for 2 seconds and contract your chest muscles to repeat above.

Push-Ups and/or Dips: Bang out a bunch as fast as you can and perform the last few by going down slowly, blasting up and squeezing pecs on top 2-3 seconds.

Legs:

Back Leg Curl: Flexed Feet (toes pulled forward toward bench). Explode up, hold and squeeze hamstrings 2-3 seconds. Let down slowly and get full extension. NOTE: Best to always extend with back leg curl and get full range of motion. You can perform a few with partial extension (pulsing), but you should always perform most with full extension.

Leg Extension: Always proceed with caution. Skip this machine if you have prior knee injuries. For the rest of you, keep feet flexed (toes toward your face) at ALL TIMES. Explode up and hold on top while squeezing quads 2 to 3 seconds (make sure you don't over extend to prevent injury to patella and meniscus). Lower slowly and repeat after feet get slightly above 90 degrees which means don't let your heels go under the seat.

Back:

Low Row: Grab a V-Bar or straight bar (hands shoulder width). Keep knees slightly bent and locked. Pull the V-Bar into your chest. Pull elbows behind you, and pop chest forward while squeezing in between shoulder blades with V-Bar or squeezing Your lats when pulling a straight bar for 2 to 3 seconds. Release slowly until arms are extended in front of you. Try to extend your arms and don't just lean forward to release the weight. This is not a lower back exercise. You are using your biceps, lats, rhomboids and traps. You can vary it up by pulling bars high on chest or lower above the navel. Best to keep shoulder neutral. (Don't pull the weight while traps and shoulders are elevated toward your ears.)

Wide Grip (full grip, back hand facing you, hold at bend of bar) / Close Grip Pulls (palms facing you/ hands 4-6 inches apart): Wide Grip – Lean back and pull down high on chest and squeeze your lats and in between shoulder blades for 2-3 seconds. Let up slowly. Extend at top and repeat. Second method – sit erect and hold same way but lean slightly back just enough for bar to almost skim your nose as you pull down under your chin like doing a chin-up. Never pull the bar down below your chest level.

One Arm Row: Square up in a three-point stance with shoulders and hips square. Your hand should be in front and at hip level so you're bent over with your shoulders slightly higher than your hips and your back is straight but not sloped. Pull the dumbbell from a full extension up until your elbow is above your back level. Hold up on top and squeeze both your lat and back of shoulder area for 2 to 3 seconds. Lower slowly and repeat.

Note: Most common stance – place one knee on the bench along with the same side hand and extend the weight with the opposite hand (same side as the leg on the ground behind your hips in slightly bent position).

Pull-Ups (close grip, wide grip, narrow grip, v-bar, horizontal bars) Perform a pull-up and hold on top 3-20 seconds to change things up and let yourself down slowly with resistance. Pause at the bottom and fire up. If you can't perform a pull-up, hold onto bar and jump off the ground so you can hold yourself up with your chin over the bar (hold under grip and over grip) for as long as you can. Also, jump up off the ground and lower yourself halfway. Hold yourself in position as long as you can.

Shoulders:

Bent over Raises: Sit on the edge of the bench. Lean over with two dumbbells hanging below your thighs (behind knees). Lean slightly forward but make sure your back is straight and head looking slightly down. Bend elbows slightly and lock in position. Raise dumbbells until you can't go any farther. Squeeze your rhomboids (between shoulder blades) for 2 to 3 seconds. Lower slowly and repeat.

Shoulder Press: Standing or sitting on the edge of the bench. Hold a dumbbell in each hand. Elbows should be at shoulder level. Press straight up and squeeze your shoulders on top for 2 to 3 seconds. Lower slowly and repeat. Don't bring the dumbbells together on top.

Abs:

Hanging leg Raises: Draw knees up high to chest and hold up on top for 2 to 3 seconds. Obliques: keep knees bent and together. Shift legs and hips to one side (right side example). Bring shins up toward right side of body and hold 2 to 3 seconds while squeezing abs and lower slowly. Repeat for 5-20 reps and Repeat for left side.

X-Leg Crunches: Cross your ankles and keep knees wider than hip distance. Knees should be slightly forward with hands on ears and elbows wide. Your chin should be an inch from your chest with your upper back off mat. You should be looking over your knees the entire time. Flex abs and hold 2 to 3 seconds, then release slightly to starting position. Don't release tension and never let chin snap back.

Bicycle: Start in crunch position with bent legs and feet pointed. Your elbows should be out wide with your hands on your ears. Bring your right elbow over toward the floor as you bring your left elbow over to your bent right knee. Your left Leg will be pointed and straight out 30 to 45 degrees. Make sure your toe is pointed. Squeeze abs entire time, but once elbow almost taps the opposite knee, hold on top squeeze 2 to 3 seconds. Repeat opposite side.

Arms:

Bicep Straight Bar Curls: Start with a 25 lb. straight bar and your feet shoulder distance apart. Your hands should be on the bar directly in front of your shoulder. (When you bring the bar up, your hands shouldn't be lateral to your shoulders.) Squeeze your bicep and pull bar up toward your chest or vary it up by pulling up so the bar hits the bridge of your nose. At top squeeze your biceps 2 to 3 inches. Let down slowly for full extension and repeat. See variation reps later in the book.

Close Grip Bar Press: Lie on a bench with hands slightly narrower than shoulders. (Hands 2 inches apart will add too much stress on your wrists.) Lower slowly to mid chest and press hard. Squeeze triceps on top 2 to 3 seconds. Let down slowly and repeat.

HABIT: Hold the moment is a great way to mix up your workouts.

TIP: This method is great for building muscular endurance.

SHORTCUT: Go heavy and have a spotter help you hold the weight or you up (pull-ups, push-ups) for longer period of time.

BOTTOM-LINE: Holding a contraction can help stimulate muscle growth.

9

FITNESS ACTION NO. 9

PULSE IT

Pulsing is a great way to make those muscle fibers grow and get that extra burn. You shouldn't do this every workout, but using this method once a week is a great way to get more out of your workout. The only way to do pulsing is at the end of a set when the muscle you're working is fatigued. It works best with cable machines or dumbbells but will work with a straight bar too.

Method: Lift heavy for 5-8 reps. The last rep should be almost your failure point. Drop the weight slightly so you can pulse the same motion 2 to 4 inches for another 10 reps or keep the same weight and pulse for another 5 reps. HOLD your very last rep for 2-5 seconds and squeeze the muscle being trained.

By the way, this works great for standing or sitting calf raises.

See below Exercises for Each Body Part to Pulse:

Biceps:

Cable Curls: straight bar, one handle, EZ curl bar, rope: **pulse at top**

Dumbbells: concentration curls, hammer curls, bicep curl: **pulse at top**

Straight Bar Curl: bicep curl: **pulse at top**

Triceps:

Cable Machine: standing or kneeling push downs (rope, straight bar, one handle): **pulse at bottom.**

Dumbbells: kickbacks, overhead extensions (one and two arm): **pulse at top**

Bar: tricep close grip bench press, nose breakers: **pulse at top**

Legs:

Back Leg Curl Machine (standing, sitting, prone): **pulse at top**

Front Leg Curl Machine: toes always flexed (3 ways: feet straight, heels together toes out, toes in heels out): **pulse at top**

Bar: squats (squatting on lower position with light weight only): **pulse at bottom**

Dumbbells: front squat with one dumbbell, stationary lunges: **pulse at bottom**

Fitness Ball: back leg supine curls: **pulse at flexion (ball is drawn in)**

Chest:

Machines: press (sitting, lying): **pulse at end of movement (extension)**

Bar: Flat and incline press **pulse at top**

Dumbbells: flat, decline and incline press/ flat, decline and incline flies: **pulse at top and on bottom of fly.**

Shoulders

Machines: shoulder press (sitting), cable (straight bar, one handle, rope): **pulse at top**

Bar: shoulder press standing: **pulse at top**

Dumbbells: shoulder press, side raises, front raises, bent over raises: **pulse at top**

Calves TIP (perform 3-6 sets with feet in following positions 1. put feet straight hip distance 2. feet with toes in touching and heels out 3. toes out and heels in touching).

Machines: standing, sitting calf machines, leg press with locked knees: **pulse at top**

Dumbbells: standing on edge holding a support and holding one dumbbell in hand of calf you are training (stair, wedge, etc.): **pulse at top**

Back:

Machines: pull down (bar): wide grip, close grip, seated cable rows: **pulse at chest**

Bar: T-Bar rows: **pulse at top**

Dumbbells: one arm rows, two arm rows (standing, leaning over 45 degrees) palms up: **pulse at top**

HABIT: Work these into your routine once per week.

TIP: Squeeze your muscle being trained throughout pulses and hold each rep for 2 seconds and the last rep for the longest 3-5 seconds. **Combine full reps, half reps (see below) and pulses.**

Example: Low Row Cable Machine: Perform 5 to 8 full reps immediately followed by 4 half reps (see FITNESS ACTION #10) immediately followed by 6 pulses and hold last rep with good form 3-5 seconds (squeezing back muscles).

SHORTCUT: Train with a buddy to help you get some heavier pulses at the end of your set.

BOTTOM-LINE: Pulses will help stimulate muscle growth.

10

FITNESS ACTION NO. 10

HALF IT

Performing half reps is just like the pulsing method, but you're doing half a rep rather than pulsing a small range of motion (2 to 4 inches).

You should do half pulses after you've completed at least 5 to 8 heavy reps. You can use the same weight.

Below are some of the basic exercises and movements that work best for half reps.

Bench (use a spotter): Go from chest to halfway up and repeat and/or go halfway down and back up to top. Last rep hold at halfway point for 2-5 seconds.

Straight Bar or Dumbbell Curls: Go from your legs to halfway up and/or from top to halfway down and repeat. Last rep hold at half point for 2-5 seconds.

Close Grip Presses (triceps): Go halfway down and back up to top. Skip from the bottom half as you may injure your shoulder. Last rep hold at half point for 2-5 seconds.

Tricep Push Downs: Push down from waist level to legs and/or from chest to waist level.

Last rep from waist level to legs hold at legs for 2-5 seconds. Last rep from chest to waist level hold at waist level for 2-5 seconds.

Back Pull Downs (wide and close grip): Start halfway up from top and bring to chest. Bring back up to half way point and back to chest. Repeat. Last rep hold at chest for 2-5 seconds.

Leg Press: Start from halfway up and bring to bottom (make sure you never roll your lower back off the support) and/or from top go halfway down and repeat. On the last rep, hold at halfway point for 2-5 seconds and return to top.

HABIT: Work these into your routine once per week.

TIP: Combine half reps with pulsing reps (see pulsing tip above). Don't over use. Hold last rep for as long as you can or 2-5 seconds at the midpoint of your full rep (isometric contraction) on certain exercises (i.e., straight bar curl, shoulder press, front raise...) and the contraction point (concentric contraction i.e., low row, one arm row...).

SHORTCUT: Train with a buddy to help you get more half reps at a heavier weight.

BOTTOM-LINE: Half reps will help stimulate muscle growth.

11

FITNESS ACTION NO. 11

CARDIO ON AN EMPTY STOMACH

Look. You've probably read this at least once. "Run or walk when you first wake up to burn more fat!"

In college, I studied biochemistry and nutrition. The nutritional science has not changed much in the last twenty-five years.

Many proponents say fatty acids will not be utilized to the levels needed to create fat loss from your belly due to the uptake of the body's ability to create sugars from amino acids. Look, this is true because nutritional science is like any other science — based upon facts and microscopic analysis of cell activity at all levels. However, based upon my own experiences when I had to drop 15-25 lbs. every wrestling season, I found that this would burn those extra pounds off my body.

There are both pros and cons to this so-called "training in a fasting state." Your fatty acids are more prevalent in your blood when your body is in a "fasting state" first thing in the morning. Many who don't use this method will say that in order to burn these fatty acids as fuel, you have to train in an aerobic state for at least an hour or go beast mode for thirty minutes (sprinting, hill sprinting, stair sprinting, heavy bag hitting, etc.).

Yet, I'll go out on a limb and say that since the blood lipid levels are increased during fasting after waking, your body is going to use a portion of them for fuel, even if small amounts. If you eat a meal concentrated in sugars, complex or not, your body will utilize them as your primary energy source. Many times if you eat them too close to training, you can cramp and get a very uneven flow of blood sugar levels resulting in both dizziness and weakness.

So, cut through the bullshit. You will burn more fatty acids if you haven't eaten anything in the last six to eight hours.

Remember, you're doing this to lose weight. If you're trying to make gains. Don't do this.

My advice:

If you're trying to lose a few pounds. Try it. Just make sure you're not diabetic or hypoglycemic. Also, if you're used to eating a stack of pancakes, replace your pancakes with an orange for at least 2-3 sessions prior to doing cardio. Most importantly, DON'T cut out all your sugars on the very first day of training without any food or even the first week of training. Build up your cardio so your body can adapt to regulating bloods sugars.

Certainly don't do this if you're training for a triathlon or competition that requires a surplus of sugars as fuel.

You can be your own study.

WARNING: If don't eat a lean diet for the rest of the day, then FUCK IT. You can't expect this to work if you go stuff yourself with a glazed donut or a blueberry muffin after you use this method. See later in the book for the best diet to eat.

This is definitely not for:

- Body Builder
- Diabetic or Hypoglycemic person
- Elite Runner, Triathlete, etc.
- Person who doesn't give a fuck about losing weight.
- Power Lifter

This might be an option for:

- Frustrated with no weight loss
- Serious and motivated to lose weight
- Willing to try for at least a week or two.

My Final Opinion: I used this to drop 15-20 lbs. every wrestling season in college and have had clients use it who have had seen stubborn weight drop off.

Suggested Post-Cardio Meal: Protein with carbs.

2 Examples:

1. Smoothie

    Blend until smooth: 3/4 cup frozen pineapple (helps protein digestion), ½ banana (somewhat ripe), 1 cup unsweetened coconut/almond milk, ¼ cup quick natural oats, 2 scoops favorite natural whey or hemp protein and a scoop of powdered branched chain aminos to replace any aminos that were used as an energy source.

2. 4-5 Scrambled Egg whites, 2-3 slices organic turkey bacon and a slice of Ezekiel toast. Branched chain amino supplements.

HABIT: Try it every day for a week or two. Use it only to drop some weight.

TIP: Once you get to a goal weight, start incorporating some food prior to training. Hence, the more fuel you have, the more intense your training can be. Make sure to choose a fast-acting carb your body can utilize. I don't suggest ingesting a high protein and/or fatty meal.

SHORTCUT: Increase your amino acid levels by mixing an amino supplement and water thirty minutes prior to training.

BOTTOM-LINE: I brought this topic up because I hear it all the time. I would suggest you use this only unless you've tried everything to lose weight and failed. I'd rather you change your eating habits and activity level. Work on living a healthier life and fuck the tricks and one shot tips that are temporary. This is only to get you motivated. Train and eat healthy forever.

COACHEDFITRX.COM

12

TAKING ACTION NO. 12

PERFORM 15-MINUTE WORKOUTS EVERY DAY

You should be training every day unless you have a serious injury, medical condition or simply don't care. There is no excuse that you can't do something at least every day for fifteen minutes. You won't get ripped or even be in optimum shape. However, it's better than nothing. You can find fifteen minutes in your day. Pair it up with a lean diet and wham — you may look like George Michael.

15 Minute Workout Schedule for Beginner and Advanced Level

You can pick a body weight exercises or weight plan. Below I've given you both to choose from. If you want, you can perform 2-3 sets of body weight exercises and 2-4 sets of heavy weight exercises below or vice versa.

Beginner

<u>Body Weight and Cardio</u> Workout:

Monday, Wednesday and Friday.

Perform 10 of each body weight exercise below and repeat all for 3 minutes, no rest. Rest 2 minutes and Repeat the same program 2 more times.

3 x (5 exercises below x 10 reps all repeat for 3 minutes, no rest)

Body Weight Exercises to use for above:

1. Push-Ups
2. Pull-Ups
3. Squats
4. Jumping Squats
5. Crunches

Tuesday, Thursday, Saturday.

Perform each cardio Exercise Below for 30 seconds. Rest 1 minute and repeat 2 more times.

Cardio Exercises: Running High Knees in place, Skaters, Punching, Jump Rope, Burpees or Jumping Jacks with a fist.

NOTE: Days of the week

Advanced

<u>Body Weight and Cardio</u> Workout:

Monday, Wednesday and Friday.

Perform 20 of each body weight exercise above (1 to 5) and repeat all for 4 minutes, no rest. Rest 1 minute and repeat the same program 2 more times.

4 x (5 exercises above x 20 reps all repeat for 4 minutes, no rest)

Tuesday, Thursday, Saturday.

Perform each cardio exercise below for 1 minute and repeat 1 more time with no rest.

Cardio Exercises : Running High Knees in place, Skaters, Punching, Jump Rope, Burpees or Jumping Jacks with a fist.

You Want to Use Weights Instead?

Please note that these workouts are <u>for 15 minutes! You'll go from one exercise to the next without rest as numbered and circuit 2-3x (beginner) or 3-5x (advanced).</u>

Beginner

<u>Weight</u> and <u>Cardio</u> Workout:

<u>Tuesday, Friday</u>

Perform 2-3 sets of each exercise below for 6 to 10 reps, heavy (65%-80% max rep)

*perform the dead lift one day per week, Friday (make sure good form with a belt and never with a weak lower back).

Weight Exercises for Above Programs:

1. Flat Bench (bar)
2. Squats
3. Straight Bar curls
4. Dead lifts (only 1 day per week — Friday)
5. Shoulder Press (bar) 6. Shrugs

<u>Sunday</u>

Perform 2-3 sets of each exercise below for 12 reps, lighter (50%-60% max rep).

1. Incline Bench (dumbbells)
2. Upright Rows (bar)
3. Alternate Lunges with Dumbbells 12 each leg
4. Close Grip Tricep Press, bench (bar)
5. Bent Over Raises (dumbbells)

Monday, Thursday, Saturday

Cardio: Running High Knees in place, Skaters, Punching, Jump Rope, Burpees or Jumping Jacks with a fist.

Beginner: Perform each for 1 minute and repeat for 3 minutes. Rest 1-2 minutes and repeat 2 more times with a minute rest between each program circuit.

Advanced

Weight and Cardio Workout:

Tuesday, Friday

Perform 3-5 sets of each weight exercise below 3 to 8 reps, heavy (75-90% max rep)

1. Flat Bench (bar)
2. Squats
3. Straight Bar curls
4. Dead lifts (only 1 day per week — Friday)
5. Shoulder Press (bar)
6. Shrugs

Monday, Wednesday, Saturday.

Perform each cardio exercise below for 1 minute and repeat 1 more time with no rest.

Cardio Exercises: Running High Knees in place, Skaters, Punching, Jump Rope, Burpees or Jumping Jacks with a fist

Or sprint 7 minutes out and 7 minutes back.

Sunday

Perform 2-3 sets of each weight exercise below for 10-15 reps, lighter (60%-70% max rep). Skip Deadlifts.

1. Incline Bench (dumbbells)
2. Upright Rows (bar)
3. Alternate Lunges with Dumbbells 12 each leg
4. Close Grip Tricep Press, bench (bar)
5. Bent Over Raises (dumbbells)
6. One Arm Rows (dumbbells, 5 reps per arm, heavy weight, followed immediately by chin ups till failure).

HABIT: Use your body as your gym for at least 15 minutes everyday

TIP: Buy a set of dumbbells (10, 15, 20 lbs.). Mix up the resistance days by doing pull-ups and/or dips with a dumbbell laced between your feet. Add in more complex exercises like a squat and press and/or curl and press. Now you're doing 2 exercises in 1 and cutting time.

SHORTCUT: Make your workouts simple if you can't make it to the gym and daily do 5 of each: push-ups, pull-ups and squat for the first 10 minutes and then jump rope or jumping jacks along with jumping squats for the last 5 minutes.

BOTTOM-LINE: Don't let time be an excuse not to workout.

13

FITNESS ACTION NO. 13

TRAIN YOUR LEGS

Guys. Believe me. If you're trying to look good for the ladies, you've got to train your legs. Your legs and hips are your powerhouse. There isn't an athlete (at least in a tough sport) who doesn't have powerful hips and legs. It's simple. Basic exercises are all it takes to get strong, great legs. Now, you don't necessarily have to use a lot of weights, if you don't want large legs. You can simply stick with just squats with and without weight plus sprints and jump rope. Make the effort and train legs at least once a week. If you do train legs only once a week, train them with heavy weights.

Warning: slowly build them up over time (3 to 6 weeks) to train heavy. Add heavier weight in small increments.

MASTER LEG DEVELOPER = THE SQUAT

There are different squats that you can perform: Front Bar Squat, Smith Machine Squat, Low Bar or High Bar Squat, Dumbbell Squat... The squat can be a science on its own. I'd rather not get into the technicalities of the squat as this would be a book in itself. However, if you are not a powerlifter who can build up to a low bar or high bar squat. I'd recommend using a single dumbbell to perform a squat to prevent less injury to your knees, lower back, wrist and abdominal cavity (hernia).

Here is My Squat Technique for a single dumbbell but could be used with a low or high bar technique:

Simply, hold a dumbbell horizontal within the palm of your hands under your chin tight to your chest. Belt optional but recommended. Feet little more than hip width apart, turn your toes slightly out (natural for your anatomical knee and hip range). Breathe in and tighten up your abdominal wall to support your lower back. Best to keep breadth entire time with heavy weight. To start squat, drive your hips back and slightly lean forward as you push all weight back on heels going back. On bottom position, butt slightly lower then knees or parallel to knees (Knees should be driven where your toes point in track with feet, not over toes). Pressing up, throw hips forward and squeeze glutes and keep chin slightly up. Looking forward is fine if you're a good at squat. Lock out on top and breathe out. Start over.

NOTE: a taller person will have a slightly different approach to squatting to keep a neutral spine. Never round your back during a squat which usually happens at the midpoint of the squat. For a low or high bar squat, I recommend using wrist wraps with heavier weight.

Again, consult a professional powerlifter to get the best squatting technique for your body.

PHASE 1, Leg Workout (BEGINNER)

MISSION: increase muscle endurance. Condition inner thighs, quads and hamstrings.

DAY 1 / DAY 4 (week 1-4):

Perform all exercises # 1 to #6 below and rest 1 minute.

Repeat 2 more times for a total of 3 sets.

1. Squat with no weight 25 Reps
2. Jumping Squat with no weight 10 reps
3. Skating 30 seconds
4. If at the gym: Leg Press 10 reps (50% max). If At Home: Walking Lunges 40 feet with no weight
5. If at the gym: Back Leg Curl Machine 15 reps (40% max). If At Home: Stiff Leg Dead Lifts
6. Jump Rope 1 minute

Rest 1 Minute and repeat the entire program #1 to #6 again, 2 more times.

PHASE 2, Leg Workout (BEGINNER)

MISSION: increase muscle endurance and strength. Condition legs.

How to do: perform each exercise and then its complimentary Active Rest. Stay on each exercise and finish all reps before proceeding to the next exercise. Example: perform 1 set x 12 reps of squats then immediately do 50 crunches and stretch for 2-3 minutes. Perform the next set and repeat until done with all 3 sets. Then go on to exercise 2 with its complimentary Active Rest.

NOTE: For your convenience, I've added different exercises dependent if your lifting at home or the gym.

1 / DAY 4 (week 5-8):

1. ***Squat with dumbbell or bar**

   -Warm up Set 1 x 15 reps (dumbbell 40% max, bar with light weights, 30% max)

   -3 sets x 12 Reps (dumbbell @60% max, bar @50-60% max)

   *Example:12 reps @60% max. If your max weight for 1 squat rep with the bar is 185 lbs (45lb. bar + two 25 lb. plates, 1 on each side). You'll do 60% of 185lbs. for 12 reps, 111lbs. You can't add this weight to the bar so you'll round up to the closest weight to add to the bar. Hence, you'll add two 35 lb. plates to a 45lb. bar, 115 lbs.

   Active Rest 2-3 minutes in between squat sets (stretch hamstrings and quads **plus do 50 crunches.**)

2. **Jumping Squat holding a 10-20 lb. medicine ball**

   -3 sets x 10 reps

   Active Rest 1 minute in between Jumping Squats stretch your hamstrings and quads **plus do 10-30 leg lifts, see fit action #24 for technique.**

3. **If at the gym:**

    Leg Press

    2 sets x 15 reps (50% max)

4. **If at Home:**

    Walking Lunges

    2 sets x 40 feet holding 10-15lbs dumbbell in each hand.

    Active rest 2-3 minutes in between leg press or walking lunges and perform 1 minute of abs or another body part your working on i.e. Arms: straight bar curls

5. **If at the gym:**

    Back Leg Curl Machine

    3 sets x 10 reps (60% max)

6. **If At Home:**

    Stiff Leg Dead Lifts with dumbbells

    3 sets x 12 reps (10-20 lbs.)

    Active Rest Between Each Set: Jump Rope 1 minute and resume completing back leg curl or stiff leg deadlifts.

This is a progression type of program, obviously it's all based on personal requirements. Only use this as a reference as every program is dependent on your individual goals, limitations, etc.

Leg Workout : Beginner to Intermediate

MISSION: increase muscle endurance and strength. Condition legs.

(perform this workout only if you've been training legs for at least 2 - 3 months

1. ***Squat bar or dumbbell**

    - 3 sets x 8 reps (70-80% max),

    - 4 sets x 5 reps (90% max)

2. **Active Rest:** Follow the last 3 sets of squats immediately with jumping squat with a medicine ball (25 lb.) 10-20 reps.

2. **If at the gym add:**

    - **Leg Press**

    5 x 20 reps (60% max)

    Active Rest: Follow each set of leg presses with a 1-minute jog on treadmill (4.5-5.5 speed) on incline of 10 or jump rope 1 minute fast.

3. **If at home after squats perform:**

    - **Walking Lunges Pyramid**, Lunge 10 feet up and back with 10lb dumbbells in each hand, Immediately Pick up 15lb dumbbells and walk lunge 10 feet up and back, Immediately pick up 20 lb dumbbells and walk lunge 10 feet up and back, Immediately Pick up 15lb dumbbells and walk lunge 10 feet up and back, , Immediately Pick up 10lb. dumbbells and lunge walk 10 feet up and back.

4. **If at the gym after leg press add:**

   Back Leg Curl

   3 x 12 (60-80% max), 2 x 5 (90% max)

   Active Rest: Follow the last 2 sets of back leg curls with good mornings (dumbbells) 10 reps or glute ham raises 12-15 reps.

5. **If at home after lunges add:**

   - Good Mornings

   3 x 12 (10-20lb dumbbells) , 2 x 8 (20-30lb. dumbbells)

   Active Rest: Follow the last 2 sets of good mornings with 15 back leg curls using a fitness ball, lye on back and place heels up on ball while keeping hips off the ground, pull the ball towards your butt using your hamstrings, keep your toes flexed the entire time.

6. **Squat (1 dumbbell)** 70-80% max,

   2 x 20 reps

   ACTIVE REST: Follow each set of squats with skating exercise back n forth (Lean over! In a downhill ski position the entire time with shoulder forward and weight towards your butt and keep low, push left to right and right to left for 1 minute.

These workouts above are only examples and not for your personal regimen!

HABIT: Train your legs at least once per week. Best: 2x per week. Hard gainers: 3x per week — not the same workout but always include a squat (change up w/ front, back squats, heavy, light, high rep, low rep).

TIP: Combine heavy sets with lighter sets. Combine sprints with plyometrics.

SHORTCUT: If you don't train your legs, at least do the following: Squats, Jumping Squats, Sprints and Jump Rope. Heavy weight with low reps and sets is a great way to build strength without building big quads (NOTE: you must progress into training legs heavy!!!)

BOTTOM-LINE: Power comes from your legs. Not your chest.

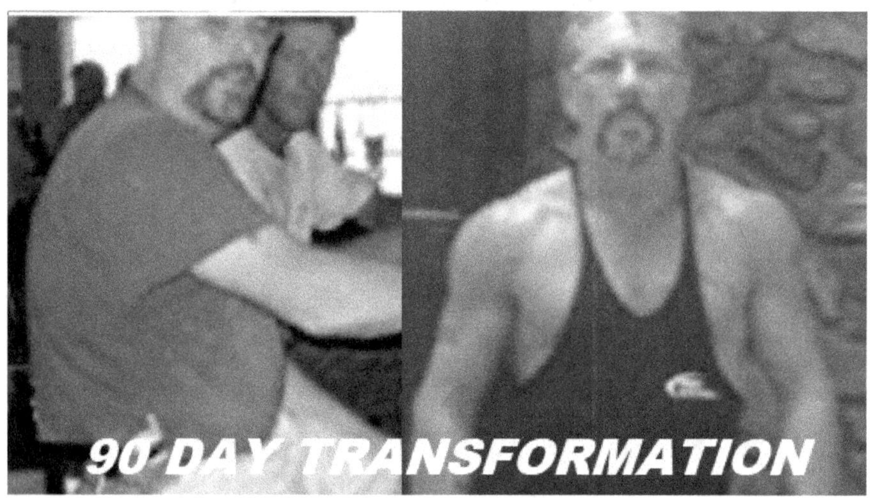

Want a 90 Day Transformation Like This?
This client hadn't picked up a weight For Over 20 Years and Was Ready To go On Blood Pressure, Cholesterol and Sugar Meds....

COACHEDFITRX.COM

14

FITNESS ACTION NO. 14

SPRINTS (THE ULTIMATE HIIT EXERCISE)

If you're physically able to perform sprints, then do it. Sprinting is a superior exercise to almost all cardio exercises to build leg muscles, lose fat and increase you're endurance (VO_2 Max). Have you ever seen a fat competitive sprinter? Thought so. If you're just looking to get the best results for your time and efforts, sprint.

However, you must start out slow before progressing into a complete all out sprint program.

I'm warning you now. Sprinting requires pre-training before integrating it into your weekly workout schedule.

Sprinting is similar to learning boxing for a week and then jumping in the ring with Floyd Mayweather. Simply, dumb. Yet, you'd probably last longer sprinting than in the ring. You must build up to incorporating sprinting into a complete workout.

Sprinting requires good muscle health, joint stability, hip mobility, core strength, leg power and the strength to work at a 90%-100% capacity. Sprinting is starting from a 3-point stance and/or standing.

If you want to sprint like an elite sprinter or you're trying to improve your speed for running, football, etc., I recommend you buy an elite sprinting program or hire a sprinting coach.

If you're just looking to get the best results for your time and efforts, sprint.

Yet, you need to do some things before getting there.

Please Note: start sprinting if and only if you can jog at least 2 miles, have been conditioning for at least a month and have no medical conditions or risk. Always consult your doctor before doing any exercise like sprinting.

Note: Wear your heart rate monitor during your sprinting training.

Minimum 4-Week Training Before Starting a Sprinting Program:

1. Basic Foundation

Week 1-4.

Mon/Wed/Fri (Circuit Training)

- Jog 2 miles
- Stretch 10-15 minutes back, legs, hips
- Plank 5 x 15 sec – 1 minute

- Pull-Ups 5 x 5 - 30 (use a support band, partner or jump off a box or the ground to get all reps)
- Leg Raises, ab exercise 5 sets x 20 reps (hands under your butt for support, raising feet pointed, bring straight legs 90 degrees to 3 inches off the ground and repeat. If you feel any discomfort in you hip flexor or groin, you should stop immediately. <u>Only perform</u> 1-2 sets for 10 reps if you never train your abs.)

Tue/Thurs (Circuit Training)

Perform #1 to #7 and repeat all exercises 2 more times with no rest:

1. Squats with bar or dumbbells (60% max) 12 reps
2. Jump Rope 2 minutes
3. Skating 1 minute
4. Back Leg Curl Machine (60% weight) 15 reps or Back Leg Curl with Fitness Ball 20 reps
5. Push-Ups 30 seconds to 1 minute
6. Running High Knee with proper arm movement 1 minute
7. Good Mornings with bar or dumbbells 10 reps

Stretch 10 minutes

Hurdle Stretch, sitting with feet wide, rolling like a ball, calf stretch on a stair

Foam Roller: side leg (IT band), upper back, glutes, hamstrings, calves

Saturday

Easy Tempo Run 1 mile: Every 2 minutes transition to a faster run for 30 seconds and back down to your normal pace.

Hill Sprint (70% max): 10 x 15-25 yards. Work on powering off your glutes and hips. NOT 100%. These hill sprints will condition your glutes, calves and hamstrings. Return downhill slowly. Rest 30 seconds between each sprint.

Sunday:

Walk and stretch minimum 30 minutes.

Now, a sprint for you might be someone's trot or jog. That's ok. This is about you.

2. Start Incorporating Sprinting

Sprint on a Track and/or field (grass and/or turf*), never pavement

Week 5 and 6

Mon/Thurs

Perform in order all #1 to #8 as written, at own risk!

1. Jog 1/2 mile. Walking Lunges 50 yards. High Knee Running in place 1 minute
2. Stretch 10-15 minutes back, legs, hips, calves
3. Sprint 4 sets x 25 yards , 75% effort, 1min rest between sets
4. Sprint 2 sets x 50 yards, 90% effort (walk back 50 yards for rest and repeat)

5. Run 100 yards (walk back 100 yards, stretch 1 minute)

7. Sprint 10,20,30,40,50 *sprint to yard then to start point i.e. sprint to 10 to start to 20 to start to 30 etc. no rest

8. Sprint 4 x 100 yards, full effort (100%), 30 sec rest between

9. Jog light for 1 mile

Stretch 10 minutes

Hurdle Stretch, sitting with feet wide, rolling like a ball, calf stretch on a stair

Foam Roller: side leg (IT band), upper back, glutes, hamstrings, calves

WEEK 7 and 8

Mon/Thurs (Sprinting Program)

1. Jog 1/2 mile. Walking Lunges 50 yards. High Knee Running In place 1 minute

2. Stretch 10-15 minutes back, legs, hips, calves

3. 5 x 25 yards, 75% effort, 1min rest between sets

4. 6 x 50 yards, 100 % effort (walk back 50 yards for rest and repeat)

5. Run 100 yards Sprint Back to start,

6. 3 x 100 yards, full effort (100%), rest 1 min between sets

7. 2 x 200 yards (touch and go) , full effort (100%),

8. Jog 1 lap, sprint long stretch of each 100 yard

9. 3x 25 yard sprints, 30 second rest between each sprint

10. Leap Frog 100 yards, 50 push ups, Repeat back

11. Jog light 1/2 mile

12. Stretch

***NEVER SPRINT 100% ON PAVEMENT.**

Tue/Friday (Circuit Training)

Perform in order all #1 to #8 as written, and repeat 4 more times, at your own risk!

1. Squats with bar or dumbbells (80% max) 6-8 reps
2. Jump Rope 2 minutes
3. Skating 1 minute
4. Back Leg Curl Machine (80% weight) 8-10 reps
5. Push-Ups 30 seconds to 1 minute
6. Pull-Ups 5-20 reps (use a support band, partner or jump off a box or the ground to get all 5 reps).
7. Good Mornings with bar or dumbbells 8 reps
8. Repeat all 4 more times with no rest.

Ab Routine (circuit 2: perform each exercise and rest 30 seconds. Repeat 4 more times).

- Crunches 25 reps
- Bicycle 30 seconds
- Rest 30 seconds and repeat both 3 more times.

Stretch 10 minutes

Hurdle Stretch, sitting with feet wide, rolling like a ball, calf stretch on a stair

Foam Roller: side leg (IT band), upper back, glutes, hamstrings, calves

Saturday

1. Easy Tempo Run 1 mile: Every 2 minutes transition to a faster run for 30 seconds and back down to your normal pace.
2. Hill Sprint (90% max): 10 sets x 15-25 yards. Work on powering from your glutes and hips. NOT 100%. These hill sprints will condition your glutes, calves and hamstrings. Return downhill slowly. Rest 30 seconds between each sprint.
3. Plank: 3 sets x 1-2 minutes, rest 30 seconds between sets
4. Leg Raises: 3 x 10-50 reps

Sunday:

Walk and stretch minimum 30 minutes.

HABIT: Perform sprint training at least 1x per week.

TIPS:

1. You can still do sprints on a treadmill though they're not as effective for either stride length or frequency.

2. Learn the proper arm movement in stride with your ankle, knee and hip movement. Proper arm swinging will help with acceleration and force.

3. Start your sprint from a standing position and eventually work into a three-point stance (you're less prone to lower back and calf injury).

4. Lean forward as you begin to sprint (fall into the sprint) before hitting your first stride. Hold your hands lightly and don't tense up your body.

5. Buy the proper running shoes.

SHORTCUT: Perform small hill or incline treadmill sprints to improve VO_2 Max and endurance. (Always consult your doctor before starting any routine like sprinting or hill sprinting.) If you don't want to get serious about sprinting, simply pick up your running tempo every 2 minutes at 70% max for 15-30 seconds. At the end of your run, perform a 90% full effort sprint for 60 seconds (Make sure you've built up your condition before sprinting at 90% full effort.)

Also, you can implement these 2 exercises if you can't sprint outside or on a treadmill:

1. Sprint standing in place with high knees (not even close to affective as sprinting forward because not a dynamic exercise).

2. Lean against a wall at an incline with both hands and sprint high knees up to waist level (imagine your legs like a piston and your knees are driving up and down in opposite direction while almost rubbing as they pass. Stomach held in tight)

BOTTOM-LINE: Sprinting is a superior exercise. Sprinting outside will give you the best results for both strength and stamina.

15

FITNESS ACTION NO. 15

LOSE THE WEIGHT BEFORE BUILDING MUSCLE

I get this question all the time. "Can I lose fat and build muscle at the same time?"

That's a loaded question. There is not a complete yes or no answer. It depends on your genetics, muscle memory, discipline, body fat, time allotted to train, and intensity, just to name a few.

So, this is <u>MY ADVICE</u> is for the majority of overweight men:

Focus on losing 90% of the weight you want to lose before working on building muscle and size. If you're overweight you've got to cut back on your calorie intake. You need to burn more calories than you take in for the day. Plus this allows you to focus on one goal at a time.

A combination of high intensity interval training and some endurance training should make up 80% of your workouts. The other 20% should focus on main lifts with low rep and 80% max weight (5 x 6 reps for one exercise per body part).

By the way, if you're deconditioned and overweight, performing cardio 6-7 days per week and adding 2 days a week with these basic exercises below, with heavier weights and low reps, will help build some muscle.

NOTE: If you have a substantial amount of muscle under the fat, then and only then can you still keep your calories higher, lift heavy and slowly burn more calories by building more muscle.

Body Parts:

- Legs : Squats
- Chest: Presses
- Back: Pull Down or One Arm Row
- Biceps: Straight Bar Curls
- Triceps: Close Grip Bench Presses
- Shoulders: Straight Bar in front of Chest Presses
- Whole Body: Cleans or Deadlifts

Your diet will play a key role to preserving muscle mass. Your diet should be higher in lean protein (amino acids) and low in fat with a few good carbs, lots of water, and a mix of fruit, veggies and leafy greens. Remember, you need the good carbs to keep your cardio intensity high. Don't skimp on the brown rice, quinoa, sweet potato, baked potato, etc.

I'll discuss in-depth diet habits for losing weight later in the book.

HABIT: To lose weight, sweat your ass off every day (6-7 days/week) and eat fewer calories than you're burning. Train like an animal at least three out of five workouts.

TIP: Focus on dropping the pounds first before adding big muscle. Get lots of sleep, stick to a good diet and train hard.

SHORTCUT: If you have two hours a day to work out, do all your cardio in the morning. Fuel up well, rest and then hit the weights hard at night. Buy an app or exercise gadget that helps you track your daily calories eaten and burned if you want to make it technical.

BOTTOM LINE: If you have a life that resides outside the gym, focus on losing weight first. Lift weights two days per week to help preserve muscle and increase your metabolism. Perform cardio to feel better and burn calories. Lose the weight. Be mindful of what you eat and live a healthy lifestyle.

16

FITNESS ACTION NO. 16

JUMP ROPE

Ok. You don't like sprinting, running or even walking. Well, **BUY A JUMP ROPE**. Jumping Rope is one of the most effective cardiovascular exercises and can be a fun discipline.

Major Benefits of Jumping Rope:

- It burns many calories if done correctly.
- A jump rope is portable and inexpensive.
- Has all the benefits of an anaerobic and aerobic workout dependent on program.
- You can look and act like Rocky Balboa.
- Heart healthy and helps your coordination
- You can use as a main cardio source for all your workouts

There's are reasons why any real boxing workout includes jumping rope — endurance, agility, footwork, speed and coordination.

I'm going to suggest both Sprinting and Jumping Rope as my two top exercises to lose weight, build endurance and get fit.

My first experience with the benefits of jumping rope was when I had a body fat booth at a health conference back in 1998. During a break, I walked around to see the other tables and came across Buddy Lee (an US Olympian Wrestler) who I watched wrestle when I was growing up. He was selling his very own expert speed rope. As we were talking, a video was playing in the background of him jumping rope. So, naturally I said, "Is that you?" He looked at me as if I was from another planet and said, "Yeah, that's how I trained for wrestling. I've only jumped roped and wrestled!"

I couldn't believe it. That's when I learned the power of jumping rope.

By the way, if you ever want to see this guy jump rope, check him out on YouTube. I believe he still sells his speed ropes and jump rope courses.

Important Learning Tips before Jumping Rope:

Start out slowly. Take small steps to improve your foot, eye and hand coordination. Don't get frustrated if you keep messing up. You will get better with practice.

Stretch out your legs, knees, calves, Achilles and ankles before starting.

Make sure the jump rope swivels at the handle.

Your jump rope should be at the proper length for you. Measure by stepping in the middle and bringing the handles under your armpits. The handles shouldn't extend beyond your shoulder height.

JUMP Roping Method

- Stand upright and stay loose.
- Keep your elbows near your sides. The action of rope swivel is with your wrist in small circles, 2-3 inches. Forearms are 45

degrees from your body.

- Stay light on the balls of your feet and jump 2 inches until you get proficient, at which time you'll jump mainly 1 inch off the ground.
- Jump up and land lightly.
- Work on form and then speed.
- Stay basic and eventually work into complex movements: shuffling, high knee running, side-to-side skiing, double unders (twice under the feet before landing), cross overs, etc. I personally only do high knee running, shuffling and running both forward and backward.

Need to see good form? Simply watch a YouTube video of Mayweather, Mike Tyson or Buddy Lee.

HABIT: Jump rope every day for a minimum of six minutes.

TIP: Buy a good jump rope and perform jump roping on a soft surface like an aerobic floor, rubber mat, padded commercial carpet, wrestling mat, etc. Make sure you wear a flexible, cushioned shoe. Barefoot, wrestling and/or boxing shoes may cause tendon problems in your foot and/or ankle.

SHORTCUT: Start out slowly — one minute for a week every day, then two minutes a week the next week and so on. Use a speed rope so it turns faster. Don't start with a weighted rope! This may cause wrist, elbow and shoulder injury. Work on form and then speed.

BOTTOM-LINE: **Jump rope to get fit.**

17

FITNESS ACTION NO. 17

BODY FAT AND AGE

Look, if you're between twenty and thirty, you're better off putting on some muscles to help your dating success. Obviously, most girls want some muscle on their guy and not a big gut. However, the majority of women don't want a guy with bulging muscles or razor sharp muscles who poses in the mirror all day either. So, if you're between 10 to 15% body fat, you're good to go.

Now, if you're between thirty and forty, you still want to look fit, confident and athletic. Plus, who really works out to say, "I'm doing it just to feel good, but I love when my belly hangs over my belt. It gives me comfort." So, you should at least keep your body fat between 12% and 16%.

If you're forty and up, you really need to keep everything in check. If you're a Weeble Wobble, you better be ready to go from zero to one hundred. Sorry but you don't have much time and you're clock is ticking. You're actually a few years from kicking the bucket. The truth sucks, doesn't it? Get over it and do something about it. Use some of these Fitness Actions (don't just read it) that I've written and you'll get going!

Remember, every year your muscle mass is dropping and before you know it. Bang! Your metabolism is turtle like. So, you'll have such little muscle that your diet alone will not help you keep the weight off. Plus, if you do lose the weight, having no muscle will make you look like a tumble-weed.

HABIT: Get your body fat checked at least once every six months.

TIP: Buy a body fat weight scale. Take your body fat first thing in the morning before drinking water or caffeine, eating and/or exercising. Many of these will give you a measurement that's not accurate but they will give you a good baseline to check against if taken with the proper conditions, i.e. no caffeine.

SHORTCUT: Have a certified trainer take a caliper and electronic measurement.

BOTTOM-LINE: Body fat analysis will keep you honest and on track. Best results are hydrostatic weighing at a university and the Bod Pod. Both are a pain in the ass and unless you're obsessed with body fat, a professional athlete or keeping weight for your next fight, then keep to a basic body fat analysis method.

COACHEDFITRX.COM

18

TAKING ACTION NO. 18

JOIN A TEAM

You loved playing basketball, soccer, hockey, tennis, etc. Why give up? If you're physically and mentally able to play your sport, get after it. Also, try one that interests you. You'll get your exercise and have fun doing it. Yet, you should try to get in better shape and/or make sure you're in good shape before starting. Give yourself 4-5 weeks to get yourself in fighting shape to prevent injury. It's best to do a whole body workout.

HABIT: Break up your week and play one day of your favorite sport.

TIP: Start out slow. Prepare by performing a whole body workout and getting into fighting shape. Make sure you play on age and skill-appropriate teams.

SHORTCUT: Work out with a small group or coach to get going.

BOTTOM-LINE: You're never too old to play an active sport (age and skill dependent).

IMAGINE TURNING BACK THE CLOCK IN AGE TO BE STRONGER, FITTER AND HEALTHIER - *FAST!*

TRAIN WITH A PRO-TRAINER WHO'S TRAINED MORE NHL, NFL, D1A COLLEGE TEAMS THAN MOST TRAINERS HAVE TRAINED CLIENTS...

- One-On-One Accountability and Coaching, App, Text, Zoom and Email.
- Nutrition Planning for Lifestyle and Goal
- Highest Level of Training Programs, 3 Phases
- 100% Guaranteed Results
- Never ask a trainer or google again and best of all...Feel and Look Ultra-Fit.

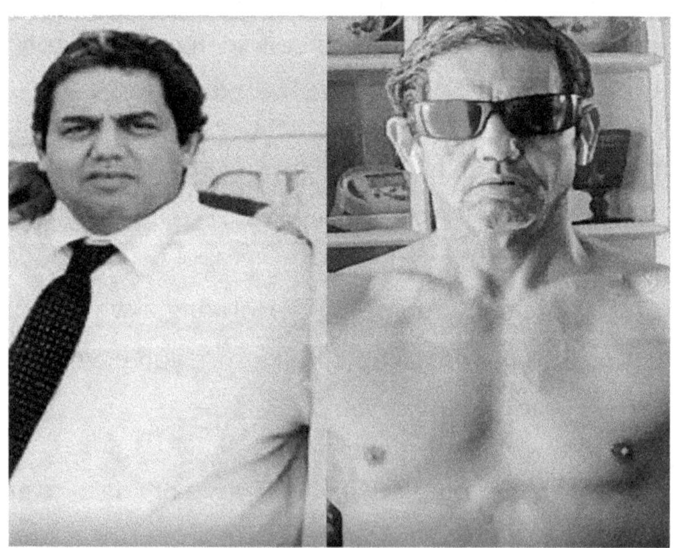

RESULTS LIKE THIS AREN'T BY CHANCE.
BOOK A CONSULT!
COACHEDFITRX.COM

19

TAKING ACTION NO. 19

KEEP IT SIMPLE

Keep it Simple

Stay on course and don't sign up for the next fitness craze. Most likely, you'll get hurt or you won't get long-term results. You are best off having a basic eating and fitness plan that will fit into your everyday life. If your goal is to look and feel better, then stick to weights, cardio and a good diet. Yes, you can add in the extras but at least keep a core program going that keeps you focused on bettering your health.

Simple Exercises for Each Body Part:

GYM EXERCISES:

Chest:
- Presses (bench) (flat, incline and decline)
- Flies (dumbbell) (flat, incline and decline)

Biceps:
- Curls: bar or dumbbell
- Concentration Curls: dumbbell

Triceps:

- Close Grip Press
- Rope Push Downs

Back:

- One Arm Row
- Wide Grip Pull Downs

Hamstrings:

- Back Leg Curls lying prone
- Standing Leg Curls

Legs:

- Squats
- Leg Press

Calves:

- Sitting Calf Raises
- Standing Calf Raises or Leg Press Calf Raises

Shoulders:

- Wide Grip Press (bar and dumbbells)
- Bent Over Raises

BODY WEIGHT EXERCISES

Chest:

- Push-Ups
- Power Push-Ups

Back

- Pull-ups (wide grip, close grip, v-bar grip)
- Rope climbing

Biceps:

- Pull-ups (close grips)
- Rope climbing

Shoulders:

- Rope Climbing
- Incline Push-Ups
- Punching

Triceps:

- Tricep Push-Ups
- Burpees down to the ground and pressing up

Legs:

- Squats
- Kicks (back, side and front)
- Lunges
- Jumping Squats
- Sprints
- Mountain Climbers
- Leaps
- Power Skips
- Box Jumping

Calves:

- Jumping Rope
- Hill Running and Sprints

HABIT: Work out every day, even if you only have fifteen minutes. Stay on 1-3 exercises and repeat for many circuits.

TIP: Don't over train. Start out slow and don't use a program from a muscle magazine. Ninety-nine percent of them were created for guys who have a good base and can train at least an hour or more per workout.

SHORTCUT: Train one body part a day with two exercises (4-6 sets x 5-15 reps) for that body part plus cardio (fifteen or more minutes with intervals of 90% max, intensity). Example: jump rope to jump rope with high knee running.

BOTTOM-LINE: Don't buy the latest flashy gadget or sign up for the big craze. Keep it simple. Training still comes down to your body, a pair of running shoes and some discipline.

COACHEDFITRX.COM

20

FITNESS ACTION NO. 20

TURN UP THE MUSIC

Simply listen to music that fires you up. Get in the moment and train hard. Forget the TV. Forget your email. If you want to get bang up results, turn up your motivational music. Remember when you watched *Rocky* for the first time and Sylvester Stallone was running up those stairs. The music made you want to do it too, right? Make a playlist that you like and use it.

Yes, I completely understand those of you who have to get things done efficiently. For example, you'll watch the financial channel while running. No problem. This is good too.

However, to get more out of each workout, motivational music will give you a boost.

HABIT: Listen to motivational music when working out as much as possible.

TIP: Get some decent earpieces that both sound good and stay in your ears.

SHORTCUT: Spotify or Pandora channels for a quick playlist.

BOTTOM-LINE: Give a boost to your workouts and fire up some kick ass music.

21

FITNESS ACTION NO. 21

LOVE YOUR BALLS

No, not your nuts. I'm talking about a weighted medicine ball. You can really up your level of fitness and strength with a medicine ball. Great for your core, arms, shoulders, back and legs. Great for sports training: lax, football, boxing, baseball, wrestling, etc.

You can use a wall or better yet, train with a partner and duplicate all these exercises by passing or helping each other. There are so many exercises below that you can literally do only one exercise for a single workout.

<u>Medicine Ball Body Development* from Each Exercise:</u>

*Although each exercise works core, arms, shoulders, endurance, etc., I've put the main benefit of each exercise.

1. Overhead Throws: shoulders
2. Single Power Hand Throw: shoulder arm
3. Lead Hand Throw: shoulder arm
4. Underhand Throws: core, arm
5. Side Throws: obliques

6. Side Twist: obliques
7. Sit-Up Position with a twist: obliques
8. Backward Throw: shoulders
9. Chest Throws: triceps
10. Sit-Ups with a twist: obliques
11. Ball Slams: core
12. Shuffle and Press: shoulders and cardio endurance
13. Running High Knee holding medicine ball: leg and cardio endurance
14. Ball Swings: standing swings, sitting swings
15. Ladder Work holding medicine ball: leg and cardio endurance
16. Toe Reaches: abs, obliques (side to side)
17. Decline Sit-Ups: entire abs
18. Single Arm Push-Ups: chest, arms

How to Vary:

- Pass or throw while moving laterally and/or forward to back, vice versa.
- Vary ball weight.
- Train with a partner.

HABIT: Perform 1-2 medicine ball exercises a day. 2-5 sets: 15 seconds-1 minute.

TIP: Form and speed are most important.

SHORTCUT: Train with a partner to push you.

BOTTOM-LINE: **A medicine ball is a great exercise apparatus** that's inexpensive and effective for your core, endurance and power.

22

FITNESS ACTION NO. 22

THE MUSCLES THAT ATTRACT WOMEN

Who doesn't want to look good? Just because you're married or have been dating doesn't mean your mate is turned on if you're fat and out of shape. Yes they love your personality, spirituality, heart, money (ha-ha), etc. But I'll tell you they'd rather grab onto a man with broad shoulders, a shaped butt, athletic legs, bulging arms and a chiseled chest. Yes, abs are great too. Yet, don't be fooled. Most girls don't want you to look like a balloon that's been squeezed on one end — you know, the Michelin Man, lug head with no legs, or the guy who looks like he hasn't eaten in two weeks with every vein projecting from his forearm. A nicely defined four-pack is fine.

So, here are some main exercises that will give you what women love. (They obviously must be combined with a healthy diet and cardio.)

Broad Shoulders: Wide Grip Bar Press (standing), Dumbbell Front-to-Side Raises, Upright Rows.

Shaped Butt: Back Squats (low with heavy weight) bar or dumbbell, Step-Ups holding heavy dumbbells, Sprints

Athletic Legs: Back squats (same as above), jump rope, running and sprints.

Bulging Arms: Straight Bar Curls, Close Grip Tricep Bench Press, Dips, Close Grip Pull-Ups, Rope Climbing, Push-ups (all variety: wide, close, incline, plyometric)

Chiseled Chest: Flat & Incline Bench Press, Flat Flies & Incline Flies (heavy), Cable Cross Overs, Push-Ups, Dips

Abs: Decline Sit-Ups, Hanging Leg Raises, X-Leg Crunches, Plank, Oblique Sit-Ups (side sit-ups on back extension or fitness ball). Medicine ball exercises, sprinting.

HABIT: Implement these workouts into your week for six to eight weeks to see a change.

TIP: Go heavy, eat lean and sweat your ass off.

SHORTCUTS: Stick to all the exercises above for each body part.

BOTTOM-LINE: Just like you, girls like to be turned on. So, if you can't change your face, hair or shitty personality, **change your body to look more attractive**. Oh yeah, most girls don't like the muscle head look. Especially when they get knocked the fuck out by a skinny guy. Sorry guys, big muscles don't make you tough (can't say this enough).

23

TAKING ACTION NO. 23

PULL & PRESS YOURSELF UP

Any real fighter will tell you that one of the most important aspects of his strength is the ability to stay strong in the later rounds (a.k.a. muscle endurance). That's why pull-ups and push-ups are both key exercises to do whether you're trying to build muscle, get in fighting shape or just stay fit. You can train your whole upper body by just varying the hand position in both of these exercises.

What they Work:

Push-Ups: Chest, Triceps, Shoulders, Core

Pull-Ups: Back, Biceps, Shoulders, Core

Main Muscles Targeted with Hand Position & Variation:

Push-ups:

- Wide: Chest, Core
- Close: Chest, Triceps, Core
- Triangle: Triceps, Core

Push Up Variations Exercises:

- Power (clapping, semi-circle): Chest, Triceps, Core
- Decline: Shoulders, Upper Chest, Core
- Walking: Shoulders, Triceps
- Pulses: top and bottom: Triceps, Chest
- Push-Up w/ Mountain Climbers: Chest, Core, Cardio
- Push-Up w/ Alternate Arm Reach: Shoulders, Core, Triceps
- One Pulse N Double Pulse in middle or top
- Power Up Fast N Down Slow
- Isometric on bottom (2 inches from bottom) or halfway position (4-6 inches from ground)
- Weighted: 25-45 lb. plate resting on upper back
- Partner: partner helps up and/or pulls you down and you resist going down.
- Push-Up on Bosu (hands on sides) to work core
- Push-Up on Medicine Balls (variations: both feet on 1 ball, one hand on ball and perform push- up and power up off ball and replace with other hand and perform push-up and repeat, each hand on individual ball and feet on one ball)

Pull-Ups:

- Wide Grip (chest): *Lats, Shoulders (Rhomboids, rear and front Delts), Core
- Close Grip: Lats, Shoulders (front Delts), Biceps, Forearms, Core
- V-Bar: Lats, Upper Back, Rhomboids, Core
- Pull-up combined with Knee Raises
- Horizontal Bars: Shoulders, Forearms, Back (Lats), Core

*pulling wide grip behind the neck can cause an injury to one of the rotator cuff muscles. Can you do pull-ups with the bar behind the head without causing an injury? Yes. Yet, no matter how long or strong you are, there's still a chance of injury.

Pull-Up Exercise Variations:

- Power Up and Down Slow
- One Full and double pulse on top
- Isometric (hold on top or halfway down)
- Jumping (sprint off floor or platform when arms in slightly bent position and down super slow)
- Tucked Knees, X-Ankles and bent knee or straight leg.
- Weighted (belt and chain holds weight between legs or x-ankle holds dumbbell)
- Partner: Partner pushes you down by placing hands on your upper back while you resist. Then helps you up by pulling up each shoulder with each hand on front deltoid. Your partner provides more assistance toward the failure point.
- Clapping behind back and in front. Looks good but don't try.

Well, I think I've proved my point that both push-ups and pull-ups have enough variations to work your entire body. So give some of these a try. If you get bored, then bob for apples while doing push-ups or perform pull-ups in a toga.

Question and Answers:

What if I can't do even one push-up?

Cry and then start performing push-ups on the stairs, on an incline, or against a wall. Also, if you can't do a real push-up, start on your knees and once you press up, transfer from your knees to your toes in a standard push-up position and slowly (I mean fucking slowly) go down to increase your resistance, which in turn will increase strength over time.

What is the best alignment for a push-up?

The best alignment depends on whether you're on your feet or knees. Knees: one long line from your knee to your shoulders. So, get your ass down and suck in your gut. Squeeze your ass if you want. Feet: one long line from your ankle to your shoulder. A line! Not a fucking V. Oh yeah, look down. No need to shoot your head up. However, you can keep your head up to build your neck muscles for wrestling, fighting, etc. or if you want to pose as a bad ass. I prefer my hands slightly back from my shoulders so my thumbs, when fingers are spread out, are in line with my armpits. My hands are 2-3 inches wider than my shoulders and elbows with triceps perpendicular to my upper body. This works the chest and the back while supporting the shoulders. You can also bring your hands back farther and tuck your elbows into your sides.

Will push-ups get rid of my milky tits (man boobs)?

Well, that may be genetic or might just be the cause and effect of you eating like a lard ass. So, eat lean protein and perform push-ups every waking moment in every direction. Simply, yes they will make a difference once you get up to hundreds a day.

HABIT: Perform push-ups and pull-ups after every workout or as a complete workout.

TIP: Push-Ups: Start out with your max repetition of a true push-up whether on your knees or feet. Then, perform that number in the morning, afternoon and night. Every week add 1-10 more reps to the morning and night. On Sunday, perform as many as you can do within a minute. Make Sure you stop immediately if you feel a strain in any area.

Pull-Ups: Purchase a thick pull-up band for assistance or train with a friend. Hold the top position for 2-3 seconds and emphasize the muscles you're training and go down slowly (resisting the down position by using your back and arm muscles). Again, fucking slowly. If you can hit your feet on the floor then explode up by using your feet and calves.

SHORTCUT: Use a Gravitron (gym), pull-up rubber band or friend to assist you with pull-ups. Keep training and don't be a pussy.

BOTTOM-LINE: **Push-ups and pull-ups can be done anywhere**. So do them. Start slow and build up.

24

TAKING ACTION NO. 24

GET A SIX-PACK

'm sure you've heard these before.

"Get six-pack abs with these two exercises."

"Build a six-pack and still eat all the foods you love."

"Get fighters' abs by just doing this simple exercise for seven minutes a day."

"A six-pack is made in the kitchen."

Blah, blah, blah...

Well, it's all crap. Unless you're a genetic freak, work ten hours a day landscaping, or simply eat very little with high anxiety. Getting a six-pack takes some dedication, a clean diet and some muscle work.

Now, you can have varying degrees of your six-pack too. Ripped and rock hard or just simply a shaped, soft six-pack.

So, how do you get a six-pack?

Well, it depends on how much body fat you have to lose. A person who has thirty pounds to lose has to take a different approach than someone who just has to lose a few pounds of belly fat.

Yet, there are some common steps to take:

Step 1:

Clean up the diet. The faster you cut out starches as well as processed and heavily salted foods, the faster you'll see a change. A Paleo type diet is the better option. Lean proteins are one of the keys to getting a six-pack. Note: overconsumption of protein will not lead to more muscle but fat.

Step 2:

Shed some weight. Many guys had a six-pack in their younger years and probably still have abs hidden under their layer of beer fat. So, you need to start burning off your unwanted fat by picking up the cardio with some intensity. Start with 4-5 days, 30 minutes of tempo-style cardio (65% max heart rate for 5 minutes followed by 1-2 minutes 80-90% max heart rate).

Great Cardio Exercise That Help Build Abs:
- Sprinting
- Mountain Climbers
- Burpees
- Stair Climbers
- Trail Runs
- Spinning

- Boxing: heavy bag drills
- Jump Rope

Step 3:

Lift heavy and choose exercises that work your abs. **Plus, the more muscle you pack on, the faster your metabolism will be and the more fat you'll burn from your midsection.**

Many people don't realize that **lifting heavy** and focusing on keeping your abs tight while performing heavy lifts actually helps build your abs. Exhale and contract your abs to engage your stomach muscles.

Biceps:
- Heavy straight bar curls
- Cable Curls with short bar

Triceps:
- Rope Push Downs
- Bar Push Downs

Legs: Squats

Back:
- Close Grip Pull Downs (bar)
- Chin-Ups (close grip)
- One Arm Rows

Chest:
- Push-ups
- Sitting Peck Deck Machine (flies)

- Flat Press bar and dumbbells
- Cable and Dumbbell Flies
- Whole Body
- Cleans
- Dead Lifts

Fourth Step: Train Your Abs

You should work your abs like any other muscle. Don't over train. Create resistance to make dense, rock hard abs (diet must be included).

Just like any other body part, training your abs depends on where you are in reference to your training program and fitness level.

Beginner **who needs to lose 12-20 lbs.**

You should start out slowly and choose only 2- 4 ab exercises for a small range of reps. Your main focus is to strengthen your core and stay with a simple routine. If you have more than 20lbs. to lose, you should increase your cardio and limit the sets of weight by one if time is a factor. Focus on burning a lot more calories than you're taking in. Yet, you must do some weight training.

- NOTE: max = max weight for 1 rep, so if you can bench 100lbs and the program reads 3 x 4 (60% max) you would perform 3sets x 4 repetitions @ 60lbs (.60 x 100).

Beginner Training Example:

Monday, Friday

Clean Diet + 30 minutes Cardio (tempo) + Ab Workout

Ab Workout: Perform each exercise (1 to 4) then repeat 3-5x

1.   Plank 15-30 seconds
2.   25 X-Ankle Crunches
3.   10-20 Push-Ups
4.   Bicycle 45 degrees 15-30 seconds

Tuesday

Clean Diet + 20 minutes Cardio (tempo) + Ab Workout with Weights (all using weight 70-80% max)

Squats 3 x 8 (65-70% max)

Straight Bar Curls 4 x 6 (70-90% max)

Close Grip Pulls 3 x 8 (70-90% max)

Dead Lifts 2 x 8 (65% max)

Flat Bench 5 x 6 (70% max)

Shoulder Press Bar 3 x 6 (70% max)

Saturday

Squats 3 x 4 (80-90% max) x 8 reps (65% max)

Example: Perform 4 reps with 90 lbs., 2-35lb. plates plus 2-10lb. plates on the bar (85% max rep) then immediately drop weight off the bar to 70 lbs., take the 2-10lb. plates off and perform another 8 reps (drop set).

Straight Bar Curls 2 x 6 (80-90% max), 2 x 6 (80-90% max) x failure (65% max)

Example: Perform 6 reps at 45 lbs. (45 lb. bar) and drop down to a 25 lb. bar and perform reps until failure for last set only.

Close Grip Pulls 3 x 8 (80-90% max), 1 x failure (65% max)

Dead Lifts 2 x 5 (65% max)

Flat Bench 3 x 6 (80-90% max), 2 x failure (65% max)

Shoulder Press Bar 3 x 6 (80-90% max), 1 x 6-8 (65% max)

*Wedneday, Sunday

Power Walk, Trot or Jog 45 – 90 minutes.

*If you have never worked out or are just starting after a long hiatus, you should listen to your body and rest one or both of the days until you build up your stamina.

Intermediate Level Workout:

Monday, Friday

Clean Diet + 30 minutes Cardio (tempo) + Ab Workout

Ab Workout: Perform each exercise (1 to 6) then repeat 3-5x

1. Plank 2 minute
2. 25 Push-Ups
3. Hanging Leg Raises 10-50
4. Hanging Oblique Raises 10 to 20 each side

5. Decline Sit-Ups with Twist at Top (hands on ears entire time)
6. Leg Raises (90 degrees to 3 inches) 50-100 reps

Tuesday

Clean Diet + 20 minutes Cardio (tempo) + Ab Workout with Weights (all using weight 70-80% max)

Squats 4 x 8, 2 x 15

Straight Bar Curls 5 x 6-10 (70-90% max)

Close Grip Pulls 4 x 6-10 (70-90%)max

Dead Lifts 2 x 8 (65% max), 4 x 5 (80-90% max)

Flat Bench 5 x 6 (80% max)

Shoulder Press Bar 6 x 6 to 10 (65-80% max)

Ab Workout: Perform each exercise (1 to 5) then repeat 3-5x

1. X-Leg Crunches 50
2. Decline sit-ups until failure (can't do anymore)
3. Decline Leg Raises with Hip Lifts 10 to 25
4. Sit-ups with medicine ball (10-20 lbs.) Hit the ground side to side at top hard so ball bounces.
5. Pull-ups: close grip until failure

Note: You can vary this workout by picking different exercises. Notice how most of these exercises are concentrated on upper and middle ab area. Monday was mostly lower abs.

Saturday

Squats 2 x 5 (80-90% max), 3 x 5 (80-90% max) x 6-10 reps (65% max)

Straight Bar Curls 4 x 5 (80-90% max), 3 x 8 (65-80% max) x failure (65% max)

Close Grip Pulls 4 x 6 (80-90% max), 2 x failure (65% max)

Dead Lifts 2 x 5 (65% max)

Flat Bench 4 x 3-6 (80-90% max), 2 x failure (65% max)

Shoulder Press Bar 3 x 6 (80-90% max), 1 x 6-8 (65% max)

Ab Workout: Perform each exercise (1 to 4) then repeat 1-3x

1. Bench Accordions 10-25
2. Crunch with kickouts 10-25
3. Roll Outs with ball 10-25
4. Bench Flutters 30 seconds to 1 minute

Wednesday, Sunday

Power Walk, Trot or Jog 45 – 90 minutes.

Perform as many sets as possible (5 reps of each or until failure). Keep abs tight entire time.

1. Pull-Ups
2. Push-Ups
3. X-ankle Crunches with heavy dumbbell

This training regimen will get you going. Below are some of the best training exercises to mix up.

Entire Abs:

- Bicycle
- Hanging Leg Raises
- Decline Sit-Ups
- V-Ups
- Star Crunches
- Plank
- Sledgehammer Swings
- Ball Slams
- Cross Body Straight Arm Reaches
- Missionary position with your girlfriend. Ha, actually works if you keep you abs tight and you're not a dud.

Focused Abs

Obliques:

- Standing Side Crunches with dumbbells
- Chop Swings
- Side Planks
- Ball Side Crunches
- 45-degree Ball Side To Side Ball Slams
- Standing Side To Side Ball Swings
- Hanging oblique Lifts
- Sit-Ups (decline and flat) with cross, cross (hands behind head, ball slams or punches)

Lower Abs:

- Hanging Leg Raises

- Wheel, Straight Bar or Ball Roll Outs
- Lying Leg Raises (variations below):
  - <u>90 degrees to 3 inches off the ground:</u> Bring straight legs, toes pointed or flexed, from 90 degrees to 3 inches off the ground, head up looking over toes, abs flexed, and hands on ears elbows out or under bum with palms flat on the ground.
  - <u>Circles:</u> Legs straight out, toes pointed, knees locked, hands on ears with head looking at toes or under bum for support with palms down, feet 3-6 inches off the ground, circle feet in to out or out to in (feet separate, go out, and come back together from up and around or bottom to top).
  - <u>Criss cross:</u> Legs straight out, toes pointed, knees locked, hands on ears with head looking at toes or under bum for support with palms down, feet 3-6 inches off the ground, scissor one foot over the other top to bottom, bottom to top.
  - <u>Flutter:</u> Legs straight out, toes pointed, knees locked, hands on ears with head looking at toes or under bum for support with palms down, feet 3-6 inches off the ground, flutter feet up and down 3-5 inches repeatedly.
- Bench Accordions: Sit on the edge of the bench, grab the edge behind you, lean back 45 degrees. Place feet and legs straight out in front of you, feet off the ground 3-5 inches, toes flexed toward you and simultaneously bring your chest forward as you draw your knees up toward chest and repeat by leaning back and kicking legs out 45 degrees 3-5 inches off the ground.

- Crunch with kick outs: Hands on ears, knees bent, toes pointed. Flex chest up and put yourself into a crunch position. Stay in a crunch with chin off chest 1-2 inches looking over knees the entire time as you kick legs out and draw them back in with toes always pointed. Kick legs 3-10 inches off the ground. If you have a weak core or lower back, kick feet and legs out higher (10 inches from ground).
- Roll Outs with bar, wheel or fitness ball
- Decline Bench Flutters: Lie back on bench with head on top and feet on ground, hold the sides of bench above your head and bring your legs in a hinged position 45 degrees from ground. Hold bench tightly and flutter straight legs (toes pointed and knees locked) up and down until abs are fatigued. Note: weak hip flexors may cause you to stop early. Rest and start over.
- Rope Preachers (cable machine): Kneel down in front of a cable machine with rope attached. Grab on each end of rope with a hand. Place hand holding rope on ears with elbows tucked into your sides. Bend at hip and flex abs to lower your head toward your thighs in arching position. Place pin of weight stack on a weight that challenges your abs after 10-15 reps and pyramid the weight down to eventually do 30-50 reps.

Upper Abs

- Bench Accordions
- Hops
- Crunch with a Dumbbell
- X-leg Crunches

- Sit-Ups (regular or weighted)
- Toe Touches (fingers or ball)
- Roll Outs

Core:

- Plank
- Push-Ups
- High Plank
- High Plank with horizontal jumping jacks (open feet 3-4 inches out then together, repeat fast)
- Cross Punching Heavy Bag
- Sledgehammer (tire)
- Ball, Wheel or Straight Bar Roll Outs

HABIT: Pick 2-3 different ab exercises and work them into your daily routine. Make sure you keep your abs tight while breathing out, etc. Hold the contraction toward the end for a longer duration as if posing.

TIP: Concentrate on squeezing your abs and keeping them tight while performing each exercise. Hold the contraction toward the end for a longer duration as if posing.

SHORTCUT: There are no shortcuts to getting great abs. It all depends on how ripped you want them to be. A very tight and clean diet is crucial to get razor cut abs. However, this book was created for guys who just want to build muscle and have a life.

BOTTOM-LINE: Work out your core and your abs.

25

TAKING ACTION NO. 25

BUILD BIGGER ARMS

Who doesn't want nice, pumped arms that fill out your sleeves? Not like Popeye, but rather like a fit Navy SEAL. Oh yeah, nicely shaped, strong looking arms are a physical attribute ladies love on a man.

First

If you're just starting to build bigger arms, you'll want to start out with lighter weights and high reps (12-20). Also, start each arm session with a lighter warmup set. Make sure you stretch your biceps and triceps. I recommend rubbing your elbows (cross fiber diagonal rub) for a minute or two at the tendon insertion. Bicep Stretch: raise your straight arm from your hip to shoulder height (abduction). Place the back of your hand on the support (corner of wall). Push the back of your hand into the wall. (Make sure arm is straight and shoulder height!) Simultaneously, turn your body away from your hand.

Second

You can train your whole arm (bicep and tricep) as a complete workout or train biceps on back day and triceps on chest day. Honestly, it depends what you want arms to look like. For those who are looking for more of a bodybuilding look, train both on the same day. Train at least 2x a week as a complete workout and add some additional arm exercises on 1-2 remaining days, example: pull-ups, push-ups, rope climbing, etc.

Third

Start each arm workout like any other muscle — with a main lift exercise (straight bar curl, one arm bicep curl). Perform each exercise with low reps and heavy weight. Follow 2-3 main exercises with 1-3 more shaping exercises with higher reps and lighter weight to get a pump.

Fourth

Train hard. Best to train with a buddy if you can. You can get some extra reps with a good spot. It's also ok to cheat a little on form at the end of each set to get a few extra reps in.

Fifth

Contract and squeeze the muscle on the concentric contraction (shortening of the muscle) and resist the movement on the eccentric contraction (lengthening of the muscle).

Example:

Straight Bar Curl: Squeeze the bicep as you curl the bar up (palm up and elbows tucked in). Hold on top with a squeeze and slowly resist the weight going down with same form. RESIST GRAVITY! Once on the bottom of the rep, repeat.

Sixth

You can build mass with a diet that has carbs, fat and protein. Yet, if you're looking for the cuts and veins, you have to cut out all foods high in refined carbs, salt and sugar. Limit your carbs to once per day and eat very clean foods without added salt. Again, it all depends on what degree you want your arms to be bulging with veins. First, get big arms. Then cut them up.

Please note: this advice is for the average guy who works and doesn't chop trees for a living. This is certainly not for the eighteen to thirty-year-old who's already somewhat fit and has testosterone at his highest levels. If you are eighteen to thirty, take advantage of it.

Top Arm Exercises

Biceps

Main Exercises:
- Straight Bar Curls: (25 or 45 lb. Olympic bar). Most gyms have the straight bar tree (pre-weighted bars).
- Dumbbell Curls: palms up (supinated), standing or sitting. Alternate curl or same time.
- Hammer Curls: palms facing body (horizontal), standing or sitting. Alternate curl or same time.

- Preacher Curl (straight bar): Sitting or standing with arms flush against a 45-degree support.

Secondary:

- Straight Bar Curl (Cable Machine)
- Dumbbell Concentration Curls
- Dumbbell Monkey Curls
- EZ Bar Curls
- EZ Bar Curls Preacher Machine or Bar
- Straight Bar Curls: Cable Machine
- Single Handle Curls: Cable Machine

Accessory:

- Pull-Ups: close grip pulls, horizontal pulls
- Climbing rope
- Band Curls
- Battle Rope Drills (battle rope exercises: double arm waves, alternate arm waves, double arm slam jumps, side to side shuffle with double arm waves, and more).

Triceps

Main:

- Close Grip Press (bar)
- Nose Breakers (bar or Ez Bar)
- Dips (especially weighted)

Secondary:

- Kickbacks
    - Dumbbell: palm facing body
    - Cable one handle: palm up or down

- Cable Push-Downs: rope, small straight bar. Standing erect or 45 degrees to ground. Press down or out.
- Overhead Extension one dumbbell
- Bar or Dumbbell Pushbacks

Accessory

- Push-Ups: standard, tricep (diamond), power push-ups
- Burpees with push-up
- High Plank
- Mountain Climbers
- Ball Throws from Chest
- Band Push Backs and Kickbacks

HABIT: If you want bigger arms, train them 2-3x a week.

TIP: Use heavy weights 2x per week and 1x with high reps and lighter weights.

SHORTCUT: if you don't have time to go to the gym, stick to pull-ups, rope climbs, band curls and dumbbell curls. Always perform band curls as an immediate secondary exercise. Example: heavy dumbbell curls 1 x 6-8 followed by band curls for 1 minute or until failure with proper form. Best short cut: swing a hammer or become a roofing contractor.

BOTTOM-LINE: **The straight bar curl and heavy dumbbell curls are your arms' best friend**. Add endurance exercises like climbing rope and battle rope exercises.

26

FITNESS ACTION NO. 26

BUILD A GREAT CHEST

Building a great chest depends on where you're starting. If you always had a great chest in college but have lost all those gains due to family, work, food or a non-serious injury, you can get a pump back rather quickly within a few short weeks. However, if your chest looks like a cow's udders, then we got some serious work ahead. Yet, the good news is that we can make it better. Not Arnold look-alike, but better.

So, where do we start?

Main Exercises (focus on these):

- Flat Bench (bar and dumbbells)
- Incline Bench (bar and dumbbells)
- Push-Ups (all varieties, body and weight resistance)
- Pull Overs (dumbbell)
- Flies (flat, incline) with dumbbells

Secondary Exercises:

- Dips (body and weight resistance)
- Hammer Strength (flat and angled grips)
- Cable Flies (all angles — kneeling, standing, etc.)
- V-Raises with dumbbells (standing holding cables or dumbbells with palms up and arms out to side, hands 3-4 inches from thighs, straight arm with palms up holding dumbbells, raise up and in until the dumbbells meet at eye level and touch as if creating an inverted V, squeeze upper chest on top)
- Decline Chest Press (bar and dumbbells)
- Machines (peck deck, isolation presses)

How to Increase Your Bench Press

1. Keep your reps low 3-5 reps for 5-6 sets.
2. Perform 90% max after warmup.
3. Every week add 5 to 10 lbs. to the bar until you can't perform at least 3 on your own.
4. On your last 1-2 sets have your spotter help you get 2-3 extra reps in after your last rep on your own.
5. Rest 4-5 minutes between sets.
6. Make sure your elbow and forearm is 40 to 50 degrees to the bar when at the bottom (bar on chest) and almost 90 degrees on extension (forearms under the bar and elbows locked out on top).
7. Keep feet planted on the ground or on a support to press heels off and drive your hips back toward your head not up toward the ceiling.

8. Go down slightly slow, touch chest and press hard while squeezing your chest, triceps and even your back muscles.

9. Breathe out while pressing up.

HABIT: Perform push-ups every day. Morning and/or night. Pick 2-3 variety and switch them up.

TIPS: Train them heavy 2x per week with main exercises and heavy weights/low reps. Follow with 2-3 secondary exercises for higher reps.

SHORTCUTS: If you're limited on time. You can perform a chest workout for 15 minutes 3x/week. Go heavy for 1 exercise and rep out until failure for 2-3 secondary exercises.

BOTTOM-LINE: A bigger chest takes effort. If you want a big chest, go for it. **Flat bench (bar and dumbbells are the winning exercise for a bigger chest).**

27

FITNESS ACTION NO. 27

SMALL CALVES SUCK

Nothing is worse than a guy with a big upper body but small, skinny legs and calves. Well, now that you know how to build up your legs. What about your calves? The good thing about calves is that you can work them with leg exercises like jumping squats, jump rope, sprinting and step-ups. The bad thing is calves are much harder to build. Unfortunately, calf development is dependent on your calf muscle insertion. If your calf inserts lower on your leg toward your heel, they will be easier to build than when inserted higher up. Yet, there is still hope.

So, let us try to build your calves.

Best Approach:

- Train your calves by performing many reps. However, start heavy and pyramid the weight as you go higher in reps. Shoot for 25-40 reps. You may have to perform 6-10 sets.
- Start at 90% max rep for 5-10 reps then keep going down in weight by small increments until you can get to the last 25 – 40 reps.

- Make sure you get full range of motion and pulse at the top towards the end of your set.
- Work calves at different angles, toes in and heels out (outer), heels together and toes out (inner), feet straight and separated 3-5 inches (whole).
- Always, stretch.

GYM:

- Standing or Sitting Calf Raise Machine
- Leg Press

HOME:

- Hold a dumbbell in one hand and place one foot behind your foot that's place on an edge of a stair.
- Sprints and Hill Sprints, Box Jumps, Ball Jumps
- Jump Rope

HABIT: Don't skip calves. Perform 1-2 exercises when you train legs.

TIP: Always warm up your calves (light jumping jacks or jump rope and a stretch) before performing any plyometric or sprinting exercise.

SHORTCUT: If you have time for only one exercise, choose jumping rope. You'll get a cardio burn, calf development and speed work all at once.

BOTTOM-LINE: **Don't skip calves**. Train them with heavy weight and plyometric exercises.

28

FITNESS ACTION NO. 28

BUILD A STRONG NECK & TRAPS

A strong neck and nicely shaped traps can be impressive. If you want to attract the women, you shouldn't build the WWF look but you should add some exercises into your training program. Honestly, it takes only four exercises to make your traps and neck look nice.

1. Upright Rows with a bar or dumbbells: Place hands 3-4 inches apart on a bar or hang 2 dumbbells in front of your body in line with your shoulders. Pull either up until your hands are almost under your chin with elbows higher than your wrist. Hold on top and let down slowly. Repeat.

2. Shrugs with a bar or dumbbells: Hold the bar hip distance apart or the dumbbells by your side with palms facing in (straight arm) and raise the weight with straight locked arms until your shoulders are up close to ear level. Hold on top and let down slow. Tip: on top perform 2-3 pulses with each rep.

3. 90-degree Side Raises: Hold 2 dumbbells in front of your body at 90 degrees with hands facing one another and elbows against your body. Raise your elbows up to shoulder height and out until your palms are now facing down. Hold on top and let down slowly. Repeat.

4. Neck Bridge (wrestling drill): On a well-padded mat, lie on your back and press your hips up into the air while getting on the balls of your feet. Roll up to the top of your head. Hands place by your ears for support. Roll back and forth and side to side.

Neck and Trap Workouts:

Training 1:

Shrugs: 3 sets x 6 reps (80-90% max), 2 x 6 reps (80-90% max). Follow each 2 x 6 reps set with a weight that's (60-75% max, drop weight pounds) and perform as many reps as you can till failure.

Upright Rows: 2 x 5 reps (90% max), 2 x 8 reps (80% max), 1 set @70% max until failure (can't do any more reps).

Bridge (lye on back, soft mat, and get up on toes and head, arching.) for 1-2 minutes

Training 2:

Shrugs: 5 sets x 8 reps (75-85% max)

90-Degree Side Raises: 5 x 6 reps (80% max) x 3-5 reps (50-70% max)

Upright Rows 2 x 15-20 reps (60-80% max)

Bridges 4 x 2-3 minutes

*Climbing rope 3 x 30 seconds – 1 minute or until failure

* Don't have a long rope from the ceiling? Hang a rope from a chin up bar and climb the rope in an L position without using your legs.

HABIT: Train your traps and neck on the same day you do back and/or shoulders.

TIP: A great exercises is to perform a shrug and then follow with an upright row as one rep.

SHORTCUT: Bridges are the best all-around exercises for a strong neck. Start out slowly and each week increase by 30 seconds to 1 minute. Max 3 minutes.

BOTTOM-LINE: **Don't forget about training your neck.**

29

FITNESS ACTION NO. 29

BUILD BOWLING BALL SHOULDERS

Shoulders are another attribute that women find to be sexually appealing on a guy. That's one of the main reasons you work out, right? If you're looking to impress your fellow guys at thirty years old by flexing your body while you grab the door, then you should probably see a counselor. Plus, no real fighter is scared of your muscles anyhow.

Yet, it's always great to have strong looking shoulders and a nicely shaped neck.

So, how do you do this?

First

If you're on your first quest to start building great shoulders, you'll want to start out with weights (50% max), low rep 8-10 and 2-4 sets. Make sure you stretch your shoulders.

A Few Stretches:

- Circling arms forward and backward 10-20 each
- Holding onto a support and leaning back while placing your head down (relaxed) and slowly stretching the front and back of shoulders.
- Pulling straight arm across your body, under your chin and reaching to the opposite shoulder's scapula.
- Shadow Boxing
- Jump Rope and/or Elliptical

Second

Your shoulders are very important to making you look strong. The great thing about shoulders is that they play an integral part of many exercises. Example: you use your shoulders when you do push-ups, chest presses, pull-ups, rope climbing, burpees, etc. So, you can increase your shoulder size by just performing a few exercises.

Third

You can injure your shoulders very easily if shoulder exercises are not done correctly. Form, number of sets and the weight you're using are all important to prevent injury. Many guys hurt themselves by performing too many sets or by forcing too heavy of a weight without using a spot (partners help) or good form. Hence, it's ok to go for the burn, but make sure you are a little conservative before increasing the weight too quickly.

Fourth

Shoulders grow quickly if you perform a main exercise and follow immediately with a secondary exercise.

Example: Standing dumbbell presses followed immediately by dumbbell alternate front to side raises.

Fifth

Always hold the weight at the end of the rep for 2 seconds. Let the weight down slowly.

<u>Example 1</u>: Straight bar press above your head and hold at the top 2 seconds. Resist the lowering of the bar with a 50% resistance and repeat.

<u>Example 2</u>: Front shoulder raises. Raise the weights in front of you. Hold the dumbbells straight in front of you 2 seconds and then lower them slowly (50% resistance) and repeat.

Sixth

Your diet is as important as the exercises to building bigger shoulders. A diet that consists of the proper amount of protein and complex carbs is key for maximum muscle growth — minus the steroids.

Below are the main exercises for building bigger shoulders and the secondary exercises for shaping.

Overall Shoulder Development Exercises:

Main:

Straight Bar Shoulder Press

Single Press Dumbbell Press (Palm Placement: Palms Facing Mirror, Palms Facing Ears, Palms Facing You)

Clean N Press

Secondary:

Push-Ups (regular, power, decline)

Pull-ups (close grip, wide grip and vertical)

Rope Climbing

Upright Rows (dumbbell and bar)

Battling Rope Exercises

Isolation Shoulder Development Exercises

Side Delts

- Standing and Sitting Straight Arm Dumbbell Side Raises
- Leaning Side Raises (45-degree lean)
- 90-degree Side Raises
- Cable Side Raises from hip and in front of body
- Front Delts
- Standing and Sitting Straight Arm Dumbbell Front Raises (horizontal and vertical)
- Front Raises with Bar or Plate (25, 35 or 45 lb. plate)
- Front Raises Cable Bar, Single Handle or Rope

Dips

- Upright Rows (bar or dumbbells)
- Rear Delts
- Bent Over Side lateral Raises (dumbbell)

- One Arm Rows Dumbbells (pulling up high)
- Bent Over Raises (bar)
- Incline T Bar Machine (wide grip)
- Incline Bench Leaning Raises (dumbbells) facing bench
- Band Abduction

Neck

- Upright Rows (bar and dumbbells)
- Shrugs (bar and dumbbells)
- Alternate Upright Row N' Shrug each rep
- Bridges

HABIT: Train shoulders 2x per week with heavy weights. On the third day, add secondary exercises that use your shoulders like rope climbing, decline push-ups, pull-ups, sledgehammer swings and battling rope exercises.

TIP: Use two training days that concentrate on just Overall Main Shoulder Development exercises with 2 main exercises: 4-6 sets with heavy weight (70-85% max) and low reps (6 to 8 reps). Followed by 2-3 secondary exercises low reps but many circuits. The third day you'll select 2-3 different secondary exercises.

Examples:

Main:

Shoulder Press Bar 3 sets x 5-8 reps

Shoulder Press, Dumbbells 2 sets x 5-8 reps

Secondary:

Dips 5 then Push-Ups then 5 Rope Climbing to top and down once. Repeat sequence no rest 10x plus.

SHORTCUT: If you're limited on time but still want big shoulders than stick to:

- Shoulder Press with Bar and/or Dumbbells 3-4 sets
- Upright Rows and/or Shrugs 2-3 sets
- Rope Climbing and/or Sledgehammer Swings 3 x 30 sec to 2 min.
- Decline Push-Ups and/or Dive Bombers 5 – until failure

BOTTOM-LINE: **Straight bar press (front) and dumbbell presses are the best exercises** to building mass and bold shaped shoulders.

COACHEDFITRX.COM

30

FITNESS ACTION NO. 30

TRAIN OUTSIDE

If you have no time to drive or don't have access to running trails, the beach, etc., go to your local high school or college and run on the field and bleachers. However, if you have access to trails, a long stretch of beach or hilly terrain, then shame on you. Grow some balls. Throw on the right gear, adapt to the weather and get moving outside.

Integrate trail running, power walks and outside workouts into your schedule. I promise you there is no comparison. Running really does help you both mentally and physically. I personally run six to eight miles per day.

HABIT: Find trails near your work or home and use them.

TIP: Buy trail running or hiking shoes.

SHORTCUT: Join an outside running club or boot camp.

BOTTOM-LINE: Use your environment to train.

31

FITNESS ACTION NO. 31

TRAIN WITH A PARTNER

Training with the right partner can bring your game up 10x. You need to pick a partner who can motivate you, keep you accountable, spot you, and be part of your journey. The best partner you can choose is your girl. You can not only spend time together, but it can pay off in the bedroom, her happiness and your long-term relationship success (well, we hope).

If you need a heavy lift that she can't help with, just grab a guy in the gym. No biggie. Guys like to play trainer.

Warning: NEVER, EVER! Give your girl a gym membership for Valentine's Day, holiday or as a gift. It's like saying, "Jeez you should work out. Are you gaining weight?" ... I'm sure you know this but figured I'd throw it in, ha.

HABIT: Make a set time that works out for both your partner and you to workout.

TIP: Select a partner that will motivate you to workout hard.

SHORTCUT: Hire a trainer.

BOTTOM-LINE: Find a friend who wants to train hard and get results.

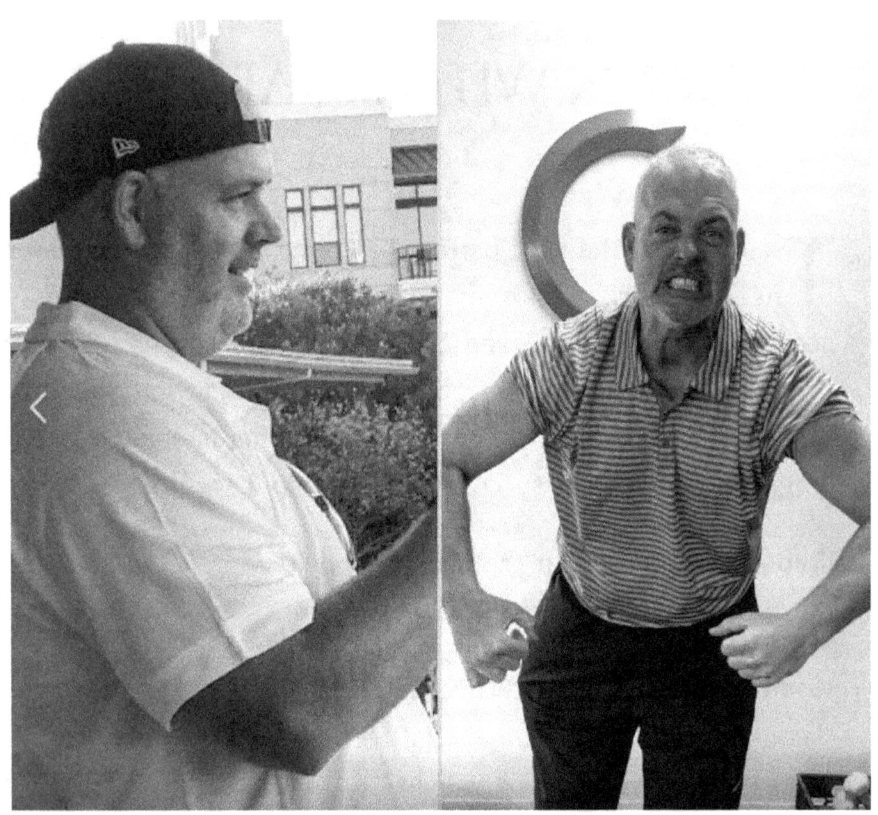

COACHEDFITRX.COM TO TRANSFORM

32

FITNESS ACTION NO. 32

TAKE A CHILL PILL

Not literally but try to do it naturally by meditating. I honestly don't have one idea about meditation but it sure sounds good. Plus, I've never even tried it. Shit, it's hard for me to deal with lying in silence during a yoga class.

Yet, research shows some excellent effects of meditation like a drop in stress, blood pressure, cortisol (a factor in weight gain) and a sense of well-being.

HABIT: Meditate any time you can every day.

TIP: Attend a professional meditation class.

SHORTCUT: Watch a meditation video or download the app, "Omvana."

BOTTOM LINE: Don't be like me. **Relax and try to meditate every day**.

FOOD ACTIONS

This section will make all your hard training pay off. Diet is the key to make or break your muscles in going from soft to rock hard, fat to fit, unhealthy to healthy. Your eating plan will depend on your goal and how serious you are about reaching it.

If you're trying to put on some serious weight, your diet will be different than the guy who just wants to drop that extra layer of fat and cut up. The food actions in this book were written for guys who want to get fit, build muscle and be healthy. If you want to get up on stage to pose then these food actions are not for you.

So, let's get after it...

1

FOOD ACTION NO. 1

CARBS

Should I eliminate all carbs?

Look, I'm hoping this book will help you make that small change for a long-term benefit. Cutting all carbs is not the best habit.

Yes, you can lose some weight if you eliminate all carbs. The initial weight loss is water weight.

Yes, your energy will increase if you eliminate a majority of your carbs.

Yes, you should eliminate all refined carbs.

Yes, you should cut carbs 2-3 days before getting up on stage to pose in your bikini. (No disrespect as bodybuilding takes a lot of discipline, hard work and focus).

However:

No, it's not best to eliminate carbs from your lifestyle diet plan (Complex Carbs).

No, protein will not give you the energy needed for endurance training.

No, you don't need to give up potatoes, certain breads and French fries forever. You just have to make them healthier and eat them sparingly.

The Carb Solution (Goal Dependent)

To Lose Weight (short term, 1-2 months):

Eliminate all refined sugars (any baked goods, all flour including wheat, etc.) Eat a complex carb in the morning and at lunch (optional). Eliminating all carbs (not including 1-3 fresh fruit servings) from your diet is ok to give your body a kick start for a few weeks. Note: Eliminating complex carbs from your diet is not a long-term solution or a healthy lifestyle. I'm not paleo and won't be. I still believe in a basic potato. I'm 45 and have fluctuated between 6-9% body fat since college without dieting down and cutting all my carbs out. No, I don't work out 2 hours a day. Not even close. I have 2 kids, job from 5 am to 7 pm with 2 hours off in the midday. I just have built up enough muscle and train 30 minutes to an hour a day.

Eating complex carbs is key for gaining muscle and not looking like a weakling. These guys you see all ripped up had already made big gains and then cut back. By the way, the majority of ladies don't like guys who look like a vein and a muscle. You might like yourself in the mirror but that's about it. Eat fucking carbs.

Morning (1 serving: 2 slices, ½ cup to 2 cups, calorie dependent)

- Steel Cut Oats

- Slice Ezekiel Toast
- Ezekiel Almond Cereal
- Quinoa
- Home Fries (sweet, red bliss)

Lunch (1 serving: ½ cup to 2 cups, calorie dependent)

- Potato (sweet, red bliss)
- Brown Rice
- Quinoa
- Frika
- Lentils (yes, they are a protein but also a carb source)

To Lose Weight (long term, 4 to 12 months):

Refrain from all refined carbs (flour, baked goods, sugar, chips, etc.).

Incorporate 2 to 3 complex carbs into your daily routine. Carb load (eat 2-4 cups complex carbs) 24 hours before any long endurance training endeavor (triathlon, marathon, etc.) to support energy stores.

Eat before and after lifting weights. Combine with a lean protein for post-workout.

To Gain Weight:

Complex carb intake is a must. Not only can it add a substantial number of calories to every meal but it also will help you recuperate and train hard for your next training session.

Incorporate carbs into 3 to 5 of your daily meals. Good Carbs of course.

Example:

EAT TILL Your Completely FULL

Meal 1

- 2 cups steel cut oats with walnuts
- Protein Drink (hemp (suggested) or natural whey)

Meal 2

- Sweet potato
- Chicken Breast

Meal 3

- 2-3 cups Brown Rice with raw nuts
- Beef
- Veggies with coconut oil

Meal 4 (After Weight Training)

- Sweet Potato
- Protein Drink with almond butter

Meal 5

- Fish
- Brown Rice Pasta with extra virgin olive oil
- Salad Greens with lemon and extra virgin olive oil

Meal 6

- Low-Fat or Full-Fat Cottage Cheese
- Pineapple

Endurance Training (triathlon etc.):

Again, complex carbs are a must for endurance training. Combine a good fat source (raw nuts, coconut oil, olive oil, Udo's 3.6.9 blend, etc.) and a complex carb 24 hours before competition. Eliminate any fats the day of competition (i.e., nuts, oil, etc.) to avoid cramping.

Must Read:

Do not mistake complex carbs with wheat. Grains that aren't sprouted can cause havoc in your body. These types of foods (wheat flour, wheat-based baked goods, etc.) can lead to gas, slower metabolism and lethargy. Example: Ezekiel Bread (sprouted grains) not 100% whole wheat bread (brown flour).

Foods (Bad Carbs) to Delete from Your Diet (at Least 95% of the Time):

- Flour (wheat flour, soy flour, white flour, brown rice flour...all flour)
- Baked Goods Including those that say, "Whole Wheat."
- Corn Syrup, Table Sugar, Brown Sugar, Brown Rice Syrup
- 99% of all Cereals and Yogurts

Obviously, you may eat some of these foods. That's ok if you lift heavy and aren't trying to get in competition shape.

A Few of the Six-Pack Carbs:

- Quinoa
- Short Grain Brown Rice

- Sweet Potatoes
- Lentils
- Steel Cut Oats
- Organic Brown Rice Cakes (Example: Lundberg Brown Rice Cakes)
- Root Vegetables
- Wheat Berry

These are all good carbs to add to a muscle-building plan. Again, unless you want to see every vein and flex your muscles on the beach like an eighteen-year-old, pick a few of these to eat every day.

HABIT: Delete all refined foods from your diet (at least 95% of the time).

TIPS: If you're trying to lose weight and struggling, limit your carbs to once per day after your heavy lift.

SHORTCUT: Buy premade frozen brown rice, quinoa or wild rice at Trader Joe's, Whole Foods or your local store's natural food Section. You can simply make a bowl with a lean protein and tasty natural dressing (marinara, spicy peanut sauce, extra virgin olive oil, fresh pico de gallo, etc.).

BOTTOM LINE: **Complex carbs should be part of a healthy lifestyle diet plan**. Be mindful of what you eat. Enjoy your diet by spicing up your foods, eating a variety of foods and making healthier choices.

2

FOOD ACTION NO. 2

EAT NATURAL

My motto since I started wrestling at age fourteen was, "If it's not naturally made, I'm not eating it." Fast-forward thirty-one years, and I'm still living by my motto. I could probably count on one hand the times I've eaten a food with preservatives or unnatural ingredients. That doesn't mean I haven't eaten pizza, potato chips or chocolate. It just means any food item I eat has no preservatives or artificial ingredients. Ever.

So you say to me,

1. "Then you must just eat body building food?"

Nope, I just make sure my meals are made from natural, clean sources like free-range chicken, farm raised beef, organic veggies, fresh herbs, etc.

For Example,

If I eat a taco, I make sure it's organic beef, taco shell made from corn not flour, natural taco spice packet (no hydrogenated ingredients, MSG, or preservatives), fresh pico de gallo or natural jarred salsa and organic natural cheese. They're simple ingredients and taste better than all the foods created with preservatives.

2. "Then you don't eat out?"

I do eat out. I'm just selective where I eat. I look at the menu before I make a reservation and/or I look online at their philosophy, reviews and mission. Luckily, many restaurants are jumping on the bandwagon toward healthier alternatives and better options. If you don't know what's in the meal, simply go for foods that are basic.

3. "What if I want to cheat sometimes?"

Then cheat. Hey, if you work out every day and you're looking just to be fit, healthy and pack on some muscle, then cheat every day. Have a bag of Cape Cod Potato Chips on Monday, slice of pizza on Tuesday and a chocolate chip cookie on Wednesday. Just make sure the ingredients are whole foods based. You won't be ripped (unless you're running ten plus miles every day), but you'll still stay fit, muscular and happy.

HABIT: Eliminate any foods with preservatives, processed and artificial ingredients.

TIP: Stick to whole food choices that are devoid of excess sugars, preservatives and artificial sweeteners.

SHORTCUT: Go through your kitchen cabinets and eliminate all foods that are high in sodium, preservatives, sugars, and fat.

BOTTOM-LINE: **Make the natural choice.**

FITNESS REALITY CHECK:

IF YOU WERE DIAGNOSED WITH CANCER OR HEART DISEASE. HOW WOULD YOU CHANGE YOUR DIET?

YOU'D PROBABLY CUT OUT FATTY MEATS, PROCESSED FOODS AND START EATING MORE GREENS, FRUIT AND FRESH VEGGIES. DON'T WAIT. CHANGE YOUR DIET TODAY!

3

FOOD ACTION NO. 3

GO NUTS

Eat nuts, but not just any nut. Skip processed nuts that are covered in oil, salt, sugar and sometimes preservatives. Always, always! Read the ingredients on trail mixes. The packaging makes you think you're doing something healthy for your body but 89% of the time...these nut mixes suck!

Yep, they are jam packed with chewy dried fruits but are covered in sugar, flour and preservatives.

So, make your own trail mix with natural, organic (if possible) dried fruits and an array of raw nuts. Yes, go with raw nuts devoid of salt, oils, etc.

What about peanut butter?

It's ok. Many people have an allergic reaction to peanut butter and may not even know it. You're better off purchasing an organic, raw nut butter (cashew, almond, sunflower seed). If you like it a little sweet, add a tablespoon of grade A Maple syrup, organic agave or local honey.

Shit, go crazy and add your favorite whey protein, smashed bananas and even some natural dried figs to it.

How many nuts should I eat and when?

Raw nuts can be a great snack to kill your hunger pains, stabilize blood sugar or add texture to your salads, oatmeal or smoothies. I personally eat them 1 to 2 times per day preferably at breakfast and midday.

Don't eat too many as they are packed with calories. Yes, good calories but they still can make weight loss difficult if eaten in large amounts (1-2 cups per day). A 1 to 3-ounce portion is good.

Never eat them before a long run or an activity that requires a lot of quick energy burst, as you will most likely cramp. If you do run marathons or longer, some nut butter the night before can be useful for long-term energy. Again, an ounce is sufficient.

What nuts should I buy if I'm on the go and I stop at a convenient shop?

Well, the good news is that many convenient stores are starting to sell raw nuts. Also, The KIND Bar is a decent alternative to any candy or protein bar. Yes, they have some sugar but what the Fuck! Stop being a baby. Workout harder.

So, GO NUTS!

HABIT: Add raw nuts to your diet. 1-2 ounces, twice a day should be enough. KIND Bars included.

TIP: Make your own trail mix. Mix up raw seeds, organic dried fruits, raw nuts and even some cacao chips (minimum) if you want.

SHORTCUT: Add them to your brown rice, salad or smoothies.

BOTTOM-LINE: **Eat 1-3 ounces or raw nuts, twice per day for overall better health**. <u>Eliminate nuts</u> if you seem to be struggling with losing weight.

4

FOOD ACTION NO. 4

TO BUILD MUSCLE, EAT LEAN PROTEIN 4X DAILY

Look, if you're trying to add some muscle, you've got to fuel your amino acid pool. Eat a lean protein with every major meal and even in between meals if possible. Most people rely on protein drinks for a quick injection of protein. However, I recommend eating lean protein choices whenever possible instead of the basic whey protein. One or two protein drinks a day is ok if you have no other alternative. Yet, don't rely on all your protein from a protein powder (whey, pea, brown rice, egg, hemp). Choose 8-16 ounces (body weight, metabolism, genetics and goal dependent) of one of the following protein choices below per meal:

Chicken, beef, egg whites, tuna (no pyrophosphate), white fish, salmon, turkey breast, turkey bacon (natural), lentils.

**Spend the extra few dollars for free-range, organic meats.

NOTE:

YOU MUST be training with a resistance type of workout (weight training, body resistance, etc.) to utilize protein to pack on the muscle. If you're not training with weights, scale down your protein intake. Unused protein will be stored as sugar or fat.

What's an example of an eating plan that's not for a body builder?

I get this question all the time. Most of my male clients who have a family and are busy creating a financial future want to eat healthy but don't want to eat like an eighteen-year-old or body builder.

Example: For A Real Client Who Wanted Some Food Options

170 lb. guy
15% Body Fat

Training: Cardio 30 minutes per day, trains heavy 4 days per week.

Goal: Add some dense muscle while shedding some fat to 12% body fat. His office was close to Chipotle and he needed options that were quick. Plus, some ideas for him to integrate for dinner that would be acceptable with his wife.

Please Note: Bulking up sometimes requires adding some body fat. So, if you're looking to add some serious muscle, you'll have to add some fat and eventually cut back on your calories. Adding fat is a lot easier to add than muscle. So, if you're gaining fat too quickly, lift heavier, cut back on fat calories, and instead add more complex carbs.

Example: A Meal Plan for a Guy who wants to add protein to his diet without living like an 18 year old bodybuilder. This is not an everyday meal plan. This is only for 1-2 days a week. I recommend limiting red meat to 2x per week at most. **Yes, you can build muscle without eating red meat or even animal meat.**

Meal 1

- Hard-boiled egg or 2 egg whites (best)
- 4 slices Natural Turkey Bacon or natural chicken sausage (no antibiotics)
- 1-2 Slices Ezekiel Toast with tbsp. raw almond butter or Earth Balance Butter

Meal 2

- 1 cup Low-Fat Cottage Cheese
- Green apple or ½ cup favorite fruit (blueberries, watermelon, pineapple)

Meal 3

- Chipotle Meal:
- Bowl with double the meat (chicken, steak), lettuce, salsa, little cheese and scoop brown rice

Meal 4

- Protein Drink or lean Protein (6-12 ounces): Sushi, Chicken Breast, etc.
- Piece of Fruit

Meal 5

- Salad Greens (kale, spinach, arugula, tomatoes) with Newman's Own Light Caesar Dressing or favorite natural oil-based dressing.
- Stir Fried Veggies (broccoli, spinach, kale and assorted peppers) Sautéed with extra virgin olive oil and fresh garlic.
- 10-14 ounces grass fed lean beef (grilled with touch sea salt and pepper)

Should everyone Eat Protein 5 times per day?

- No. Here are some basic approximate percentages for protein intake based on your goal and your activity level.

Weight Loss:

- (Short Term 1-6 months) 50% Protein 40% Complex Carb 10% Fat
- (Long Term 6 months- 12 months) 50% Complex Carb 40%Protein 20% Fat

Endurance Training:

- 60% Complex Carb 30% Protein 20% Fat

Maintenance, Health

- 50% Complex Carb 35% Protein 15% fat

Muscle Building, Bulk

- 55% Protein 35% Complex Carb 10% fat

- *WEIGHT GAIN: 45% Protein,25% Complex Carbs, 30% Good Fat

Calories will play a role in these percentages. If you are less active, you'll require less calories to lose weight. If you are very active, you'll have to consume more calories than you would if you had an office job to gain weight and build muscle. Unwanted calories not utilized for muscle building and normal bodily function will be stored as fat. Expect to add a little weight to get big gains before cutting weight to see more muscle definition.

Should I calculate the exact number of protein grams per meal and the amount of protein you need every day?

If you want to calculate the amount of protein you'll need, then do it. Honestly, though, if you eat an adequate amount of protein — 8 ounces (guy who weighs 150-180 lbs.) to 16 ounces (guy who weighs 200 lbs. plus) in every meal or even just 2 meals, you should be fine. If you want to be a nerd, then simply calculate 1.5 grams of protein per kg of weight. Divide this number by the meals per day.

However, this is only a place to start. Calculating these numbers is only for a reference point. Not everyone has the same genetics, metabolism, weight, etc...

My Opinion: you simply have to increase your protein intake if you're lifting heavy and with intensity. As long as you increase your protein, you should be ok. This means that you don't have to eat protein every hour on the hour. Since your guy with a life , you certainly don't walk around the office or work with cooler or a protein shaker.

Your body will utilize the protein it needs to make muscle period. Over a few weeks, you should be able to see how your body responds to taking in more protein. If you're not getting muscle gains than you have to either lift heavier, cut back on cardio and/or take in more protein. If you're gaining more fat than either cut back on the protein intake or increase your cardio a little. You should be able to figure it out.

For you mathematicians:

Example to calculate protein intake: You weigh 160 lbs. and want to figure out daily protein intake. 160 lbs./2.2kg/lb. = 72 kg x 1.5 g. protein/kg = 109 grams protein per day / 5 meals per day = 22 grams protein needed in each meal.

So an easy rule of thumb.

150-180 lbs. 30 grams protein/ meal (4-5 in day)

180-230 lbs. 50 grams protein / meal (5 in a day) minimum

You know what?

Screw it. Just eat lean protein 4-5x day or even just 3x per day (obviously eat more protein per sitting), sweat your ass off and train hard. That's it.

Let's Go Over the Good Protein (I'm sure you've seen this stuff 100x already):

(Buy Free Range whenever possible)

- Egg Whites (Yes, egg yolks have lots of nice little vitamins but the egg white is where it's at for protein)
- Protein Powder (whey, vegan, casein, hemp, pea, rice,egg)
- Lentils. Tempeh, Organic Tofu, Hemp (Vegans)
- Ground (organic) Meat: buffalo, turkey, chicken, beef
- Beef (flank, bottom roast, top round, top sirloin)
- Chicken (breast, tenderloins)
- Turkey (natural turkey breast not processed deli meat)
- Turkey Bacon (natural, no nitrates or fillers)
- Organic Cottage Cheese

- Natural Protein Powder (whey, **hemp, brown rice, pea)
- Low-Fat Cottage Cheese
- Low-Fat Greek Yogurt (last choice)

**Hemp powder is my favorite choice. Cons: expensive, gritty. Pros: Non Dairy, High Amino Acid Profile

Grain Sources of Protein (little)

- Quinoa
- Wheat Germ
- Frika

HABIT: Incorporate lean protein into every main meal. If you're training hard with weights and trying to pack on lean muscle, you've got to feed your muscle throughout the day with lean protein and lots of it based upon your goal and activity level. (Monitor your body fat and cut back on the protein and/or calories if your waist is not looking as you desire.)

NOTE: 80% of your workouts should use heavier weight sets to increase protein absorption. Put your muscle fibers to work and they'll reward you with hard, lean muscle.

TIP: Always try to eat organic and/or free-range meats. Keep lean protein sources in your car or work so you don't automatically eat easy-to-grab refined carb choices when hungry. **Examples for work:** light wild tuna in packets (all natural, no pyrophosphate or preservatives. Only salt and water or olive oil.), low-fat cottage cheese, homemade grilled meats (chicken breast or on bone, lean steak or fish), natural protein powder, plain Greek yogurt (on occasion only), and cooked ground meats (buffalo, turkey, chicken) in Tupperware.

SHORTCUT: Take a branched chain amino supplement to increase your intake of amino acids. I personally take them after each workout and before bed. Supplement as prescribed on bottle.

BOTTOM-LINE: **Train hard, recuperate and build with protein.**

5

FOOD ACTION NO. 5

COOK LOTS OF PROTIEN FOR THE WEEK

A successful meal plan to build muscle and/or get lean requires lean protein. Unfortunately, cooking lean proteins that are clean (no preservatives, salt, etc. like deli meats) and taste good requires time. Many of us don't have the time to cook up a tasty steak or BBQ chicken for lunch.

So, the key is to put aside one or two hours once a week and grill, stir fry and/or bake ample amounts of your favorite protein sources that not only are lean but most importantly taste good. A real meal plan should make eating fun and not a chore.

I personally use my gas grill 80% of the week all year long. The rest of the time I stir fry different meats.

On Sundays I:
- Grill marinated or herb rubbed chicken, steak, cod and salmon
- Stir Fry chicken, shrimp and fish

- Pan fry ground chicken, turkey or buffalo
- Broil or Bake chicken
- Boil eggs
- Boil Lentils

This way I always have protein ready to throw on brown rice, salad, a tortilla or simply by itself.

Most importantly, the foods don't just taste like boiled chicken. There's all the flavor without all the fat.

NOTE: I only purchase meats that are free range, organic and lean.

My Favorite Stir Fry Protein Recipes:

Easy Spicy Shrimp N' Chicken

- 1 pound raw jumbo shrimp, peeled and deveined
- ½ pound free-range chicken breast, diced
- 2 tbsp. coconut oil
- 2 1/2 tbsp. Braggs Liquid Amino or Dark Soy Sauce
- 3-5 tbsp. Sweet Chili Sauce diluted with 3-5 tbsps. water
- 3 garlic cloves chopped
- Pinch Coconut or Cane sugar (optional)
- 1 tbsp. sesame oil

DIRECTIONS:

Heat up wok or pan on high. Place 1 tsp. coconut oil and add chopped garlic. Mix until slightly opaque.

Add 1 tbsp. coconut oil and Add Chicken. Sauté until fully cooked. Place onto separate plate.

Add 1 tbsp. coconut oil and shrimp, reduce heat to medium-low, and cook, stirring frequently, until shrimp are lightly pink on both sides (about 1 to 1-1/2 minutes). Add Braggs Liquid Amino mixture to skillet; return to high heat and cook, stirring for 1-2 minutes. Add in the Chicken, Sweet Chili Sauce, sesame oil and the tbsp. coconut sugar (optional) stir until coated.

- 1 lb. free-range chicken breast (skinless), diced or thinly sliced
- 2 shallots (chopped)
- 2 garlic cloves
- ½ cup broccoli heads (chopped small)
- ½ cup organic carrots (chopped small)
- 1 large egg, 2 egg whites
- 3 tbsp. Low Sodium Braggs Liquid Aminos or low sodium soy sauce
- 2 cups brown rice, short grain (frozen and cooked)
- 2 tbsps. coconut oil
- 1 tbsp. sesame oil
- Pinch sea salt and cayenne or black pepper

DIRECTIONS:

In a wok, heat coconut oil until hot. Add the chicken pieces and sprinkle with sea salt and pepper. Stir fry until cooked but tender (6-8 minutes). Place in a large bowl.

Heat another tablespoon coconut oil and add garlic, broccoli, carrots and shallots. Sauté for 3-4 minutes until slightly tender. Place all in large bowl with chicken.

Next, place both eggs in wok and scramble until cooked. Return bowl of chicken and veggies to wok, mix all and cook for another 1-2 minutes on high while adding soy sauce and sesame oil.

Chicken Marinades for Grilling

- 1/3 cup Worcestershire sauce
- 1/4 cup extra virgin olive oil
- 1 tsp. honey or light brown sugar (optional)
- 3 chopped garlic cloves
- 1 small white onion, chopped
- 2 tbsps. fresh squeezed lemon juice
- Pinch cayenne pepper

DIRECTIONS:

Place all in blender and mix well. Keep small portion to brush chicken or pour on top once chicken is done. Marinate chicken in large glass covered pan or zip lock bag for 8 -24 hours in refrigerator. Discard marinade that was with chicken and grill chicken until fully cooked.

My Second "Go To" Chicken Marinade

- ¼ cup balsamic vinegar, organic (no sulfites)
- ¼ cup extra virgin olive oil
- 3 tbsp. Dijon mustard
- 3 cloves garlic, peeled and minced
- ½ fresh squeezed juice of lime
- ½ fresh squeezed juice of lemon
- 2 tbsp. coconut sugar or cane sugar (optional)
- 1 teaspoon sea salt

- ground black pepper to taste
- 2 pinches fresh herbs you prefer (basil, parsley, rosemary)

DIRECTIONS:

Place all in blender and mix well. Keep small portion to brush chicken or pour on top once chicken is done. Marinate chicken in large glass covered pan or zip lock bag for 8 -24 hours in refrigerator. Discard marinade that was with chicken and grill chicken until fully cooked.

"All Around" Good Steak Marinade

- ¼ cup extra virgin olive oil
- ⅓ cup low sodium Braggs Liquid Aminos or soy sauce
- ¼ cup red wine vinegar
- 2 tbsp. fresh squeezed lemon juice
- 2 tbsp. Worcestershire sauce
- 1 tbsp. Dijon mustard
- 1 tsp. dried oregano
- 1 tsp. dried thyme
- 3 garlic cloves, minced
- 3 tsp. fresh basil, minced
- ½ tsp black pepper

DIRECTIONS:

Place all in blender and mix well. Keep small portion to brush steak while cooking or pour on top once steak is done. Marinate steak in large glass covered pan or zip lock bag for 8 -24 hours in refrigerator. Discard marinade that was with steak and grill steak to your liking.

Simple Herb Rub for Chicken and Steak

Note: if you don't like spicy, omit the peppers and paprika.

Ingredients

- 1 tbsp. paprika
- 1 ½ tsp. garlic powder
- 1 ½ tsp. sea salt
- 1 tsp. onion powder
- 1 tbsp dried basil
- 1 tsp. dried rosemary
- 1 tsp. dried thyme
- 1 tsp. ground cayenne pepper
- 1 tablespoon black pepper

DIRECTIONS:

Combine and stir all ingredients in small bowl until all mixed well. Rub chickens to taste and let sit for 1-2 hours before grilling, baking, etc. Triple recipe and store for later use.

No Time to Create a Marinade?

Some Store Bought Brands that are all natural and don't suck:

Chicken Marinade: Newman's Own Balsamic Vinaigrette, Newman's Own Light Caesar, Newman's Own Lite Italian, Annie's Organic BBQ Sauce for chicken.

Chicken Rub: Emeril's All Natural Chicken Rub Seasoning, John Wayne Spice Rub, Chicken

Steak Marinade: Newman's Own Lite Italian

Steak Rubs: McCormick Montreal Steak Seasoning, Stubbs Natural Steak Rub

HABIT: You've got to keep protein at hand to abstain from lots of fast foods that are loaded with refined carbs, sugar, salt, etc. Create a schedule to cook at certain times when you have an hour to make your protein meals.

TIP: Buy a decent grill, wok and baking pan that will make cooking protein easy.

SHORTCUT: Buy pre-marinated protein at Whole Foods or a Natural Food Counter that you can simply stick on a grill. Watch out for the sodium!

BOTTOM-LINE: **Cook lots of protein for the week.** Freeze some.

6

FOOD ACTION NO. 6

MAKE YOUR SMOOTHIES COUNT

ook, if you're going to take the time to make a smoothie, get all the nutrition you can with each one. Swirl in good fat, natural protein powder, complex carbs, organic fruit and some extra nutrition.

I create a different one depending on the time of day and the purpose of my smoothie if I have one. I don't personally have one every day. I like get my protein source from fish or chicken.

For Example:

Start of the Day Smoothie:

I Choose One or a few From Each Headline **(my highlighted pics are standard)**

2 Cups Frozen <u>Organic</u> Fruit

- Banana (semi-ripe)
- Pineapple

- Blueberries
- Cherries
- Mango

Organic Greens (1-2 cups)

- Baby Kale
- Baby Spinach
- Arugula

Liquid (add for preferred blend, best if ¼-½ over solids)

- 2% Organic Milk
- Coconut Milk
- Hemp Milk
- Almond Milk
- Coconut/Almond Mix
- Coconut Water
- Water

Thickener

- Chia Seeds (tbsp.)
- Raw Nut Butter: almond, cashew, sunflower (tbsp.)
- Flax Seeds (tbsp.)
- Coconut Meat
- Organic Quick Oats, gluten free (¼-½ cup dry)

Power Boost

- Spirulina
- Wheat Grass liquid or Powder
- Green or Red Powder (as directed)
- Glutamine Powder (as directed)
- Udo's 3.6.9 Oil Blend (tsp.)

- Natural Protein Powder: hemp, whey, brown rice, pea, casein (2-3 scoops)
- Maca

Sweetener (optional)

- Natural Maple Syrup (tsp.)
- Agave (tsp.)
- Natural Dates (small handful)

Midday or Post-Workout Smoothie

1 Cup Frozen <u>Organic</u> Fruit

- Banana (semi-ripe)
- Pineapple
- Blueberries
- Cherries
- Mango

Liquid (add for preferred blend, best if ¼-½ over solids)

- 2% Organic Milk
- Coconut Milk
- Hemp Milk
- Almond Milk
- Coconut/Almond Mix
- Coconut Water
- (as directed)Water

Power Boost

- Spirulina
- Wheat Grass liquid or Powder
- Green or Red Powder (as directed)

- Glutamine Powder (as directed)
- Udo's 3.6.9 Oil Blend (tsp.)
- Natural Protein Powder: hemp, whey, brown rice, pea, casein (2-3 scoops)
- Maca powder (as directed)
- MSM Liquid(as directed)
- Branched Chain Aminos

Reasons I Personally Use These Power Boosters:

Maca powder: testosterone

MSM Liquid: muscle recovery, joint inflammation

Udo's 3.6.9 Blend Oil: MCT (medium chain triglycerides) appetite suppression, metabolism

Branched Chain Aminos: protein synthesis, muscle build and recovery

Green or Red Powder: free radical recovery and protection

Note:

If you're not dropping the belly fat then skip the nut butter and oils, cut back on fruit portions and drop all sweeteners. Increase your workout intensity and add some heavy weights along with high rep circuit days.

HABIT: Start your day with a fruit smoothie with protein, green smoothie with protein or green drink with protein plus a probiotic multiple vitamin.

TIP: buy a decent blender and a juicer that have good reviews on Amazon and easy to clean.

SHORTCUT: pick 1 or 2 favorite frozen organic fruits you like and mix with 2-3 scoops natural protein powder and liquid to blend.

BOTTOM-LINE: **smoothies are a great way to use protein powder**.

7

DIETARY ACTION NO. 7

KEEP HEALTHY SNACKS AVAILABLE

Good luck to you if you never again eat sugar, snacks, etc. Now, if you're trying to make weight for your next fight, marathon, prevent allergies, weight loss goal, etc., then stick to your goal and strict diet.

For the rest of us, keeping a good snack in the house is key to enjoying your diet.

Does that mean you should be eating s'mores, cheesecake and devil dogs? Dah.

No, instead you can sneak in some natural treats that will keep your cravings at bay and help you stay fit.

Below are my "Go To Snacks." Some may sound not so good, but remember, I'm forty-five and have kept between 5-9% body fat without training like a body builder. These may help you or you may tell me to go fuck myself. No worries either way. ☺

_________ = Top Snack Choices

- Steel Cut Oats, Coconut Milk, Cinnamon, tsp Cane Sugar
- Slice Ezekiel Toast or Ezekiel English Muffins with raw almond butter, sliced banana or natural fruit preserves. I add a tablespoon natural maple syrup to every jar of raw almond butter.
- Low-Fat , Organic Greek Yogurt and fresh fruit (chopped banana, blueberries, strawberries)
- Cherries
- Ezekiel Almond Cereal with Coconut Milk and tbsp. maple syrup
- Lundberg Brown Rice Cake with Raw Nut Butter and Natural Fruit Preserves
- ONE Bars
- Pistachios, Almonds or Cashews
- Field Greens with or without protein and your favorite dressing
- Hard Boiled Eggs
- Egg white and tortilla **grilled** wrap with low-fat, natural cheese and/or fresh pico de gallo
- Organic Cottage Cheese with berries
- Peach, Clementine, blueberries, watermelon, strawberries
- Suja Juices (premade green drinks)
- Sweet Potato or Red Bliss Home Fries with ketchup (organic ketchup)
- Protein drink

- Pears, Pineapple Chunks, watermelon
- Organic Apple Sauce
- Hard Boiled Eggs with Salsa or Trader Joes' Spicy Peanut Vinaigrette
- Cheese Quesadilla with grilled chicken (natural 8 inch tortilla, no gluten or fillers)
- Salad Greens with dried Fruit with dressing (olive oil and balsamic vinegar)
- Cherry Tomatoes
- Baked Fruit (peaches, apples) with cinnamon and nutmeg
- Watermelon with Organic Low-Fat Greek Yogurt or Low-Fat Cottage Cheese
- Apple with Raw Almond Butter
- Brown Rice Cake with Raw Brown Rice Cake and Natural Preserves
- Grilled Shrimp and Cocktail Sauce
- Natural Fruit Popsicle
- Natural Turkey, Buffalo or Beef Jerky
- Natural Turkey Bacon
- Brown Rice with favorite tomato sauce (Rao's Red Sauce) and fresh parmesan or sheep cheese.
- Brown Rice with Trader Joes' Spicy Peanut Vinaigrette or Salsa
- Protein Drink (Hemp Protein)
- Homemade Power Balls

Here's a Recipe for My Favorite Cookies (Gluten Free)

1. 1 cup raw nut butter or natural peanut butter
2. 1 cup local honey, agave or 2 tbsp. stevia

3. 3 cups rolled organic oats (oatmeal)
4. ¼ cup natural cocoa powder (optional)
5. ½ cup of chopped raw nuts
6. ½ cup of dried natural fruit (Golgi berries, cranberries, raisins, blueberries, cherries, etc.)
7. 3 scoops natural vanilla whey protein powder (chocolate if adding cocoa powder)
8. ½ cup 70% Dark Chocolate or Cocoa Chips
9. ¼ cup unsweetened natural coconut flakes

DIRECTIONS:

1. Mix the first 8 ingredients together thoroughly.
2. Form them into balls (makes about 10 - 12 depending on size) then roll them in the coconut flakes.
3. Serve or refrigerate/freezer for later use.

8

FOOD ACTION NO. 8

CONSUME A GREEN DRINK EVERYDAY

Some of you would like to just be fit and healthy. No need to build the big muscles, etc. So, one of the best ways to get a healthy dose of nutrition into your day is consume a green drink. Plus, juicing organic veggies and fruits taste great too. Fortunately, green drinks are becoming very popular, so that makes it easier to purchase premade green drinks.

How to Make a Great Green Drink:

Step 1: Choose 2 or more of the following (cup) to juice in the juicer:

- Organic carrots
- Organic celery
- Organic beets
- Organic cucumber
- Green apple

Step 2: Choose 2 or more of the following to add in the blender (1/4 cup of both) with the juice above:

- Pear
- Pineapple
- Mango
- Papaya
- Raspberry
- Blueberry
- Blackberry

Step 3: Choose 2 or more of the following to add in the blender (handful of both) with the juice above:

- Spinach
- Kale
- Arugula
- Swiss Chard
- Dandelion Greens

Step 4 (optional) : Choose 2 or more of the following to add in the blender with the juice above:

- Tumeric: Swelling (tsp)
- Ginger Root: Digestion (½ inch)
- Raw Maca : testosterone (as directed on label)
- Cinnamon: blood sugar (tsp.)

Step 5: Blend all above steps.

Need to order an array of premade Green Drinks you can add your favorite protein too?

Look online for a home delivery.

HABIT: Replace a fruit smoothie with a green drink.

TIP: Don't make it complicated. Buy premade organic carrot juice (Whole Foods, Trader Joes, etc...), Add Greens, Frozen Fruit, Good Fat and a high grade hemp protein.

SHORTCUT: Buy green drinks online or your trusted neighborhood juice bar to keep on hand for the week. They make a great quick nutritional boost to any meal.

BOTTOM-LINE: Green drinks can help you get more nutrition into your daily diet.

9

DIETARY ACTION NO. 9

99% OF CEREALS SUCK AND KEEP YOU FAT

Starting the day off with eggs, fruit and protein drinks can get boring. I get it. However, simply eating a bowl of the so-called healthy cereals found in the national supermarket aisles can hinder your progress to ripped abs. Plus, cereal manufacturers are using the keywords like "Gluten Free," "Protein Fortified," "High in Fiber," etc. by taking the regular cereals and replacing ingredients with ingredients that add negligible amounts of protein, vitamin and fiber that not only don't help to build muscle but are a waste of calories. Soy protein, whey protein, casein protein, quinoa flour, etc. all increase the protein grams on the package enough to allow the companies to add "Protein Fortified" but don't do shit for your body.

In addition, the cereals that have added additional fiber, protein or so-called extra vitamins are actually hindering your body to lose unwanted fat. Many of these cereals are loaded with refined flour, wheat, corn and rice that spike your blood sugars as much as a candy bar. Hence, they place strain on your pancreas and cells to control the high amount of blood sugar. The blood sugar caused by high sugar cereals (maltose, glucose, wheat, rice, corn, honey, natural cane sugar, brown rice syrup, etc.) makes your pancreas release insulin to help stabilize blood sugar levels by driving excess sugar into your body's cells.

Over time, if you consume too much sugar and your insulin levels are out of balance, this MAY lead to your muscles losing sensitivity to insulin, sugar cravings, increase in body fat, stomach irritation, depression and lack of energy and mental clarity.

Here are some cereals that are best:

- Ezekiel Almond Cereal
- Natures Path (bran flake)
- Organic steel cut oats
- Organic oat bran

Don't fall for the granola trap. 99% of them suck too.

Although for that go-to snack, Naked Granola (**not** BearNaked Granola) is a great-tasting alternative to the granolas packed with flour. Find on the internet.

HABIT: Don't make eating cereal a habit. It should be a treat unless it's a clean bowl of oatmeal or oat bran. For extra nutrition add any of the following: raw chia seeds, raw hemp seeds or even a scoop or two of natural whey protein.

TIP: Eat a bowl of the Ezekiel Almond Cereal or Organic Oats after a heavy training day to help restore glucose levels.

SHORTCUT: Presoak your oatmeal the night before in unsweetened coconut or almond milk so its ready to go in the morning.

BOTTOM-LINE: **Skip the national supermarkets cereal aisle.**

10

FOOD ACTION NO. 10

FOOD TIPS TO BOOST TESTOSTERONE

Have you ever bought a testosterone enhancer? I'm surprised if you said no. If you read all the marketing jargon online, you'd probably think that ingesting testosterone pills will dramatically increase your testosterone and increase your sex drive, strength, muscle development and energy.

However, I'll tell you differently.

I personally believe these supplements will increase your testosterone in negligible amounts, if at all. For example, if your testosterone levels are normal for your age and you take a supplement that increases them by say 12% to 15%, is this enough for a change? Hell no. Placebo effect, yes. Physiologically, no.

Your best bet. Ask your doctor for blood test to measure your total testosterone level. (LC/MS test being one of the most accurate.) They'll most likely do it in the morning as your T levels are at their highest.

If your levels are determined to be on the low side, there are some natural ways to increase them.

- Increase your rest and sleep time.
- Eat more complex carbs after lifting heavy or *training in a high endurance activity.
- Lose weight and body fat.
- Add a Medium Chain Triglyceride Oil to your protein shakes, hot cereals, salads, veggies or any other food you prefer. I personally add Udo's 3.6.9 blend to my protein drink and raw coconut oil to my oatmeal or veggies.
- Limit or eliminate alcohol
- Add intensity to your workouts (sprinting, boxing, etc.)*
- Review any medications your currently on with your doctor.
- Consume a daily probiotic vitamin and mineral
- **Eat healthy Fats

- *You can simply increase your T levels by not overtraining. Many triathletes will improve their T Levels and strength by cutting back or resting an extra day.
- ** Many of the diets that are on the Internet contain high amounts of saturated fat. However, this increases your calorie intake substantially, which may lead to excess body fat. So, yes eat some fats, but screw these diets that call for 50% or even 70% of your diet from healthy fats like olive oil, avocado, coconut oil, raw nuts. Instead, eat more complex carbs like yams, short grain brown rice and quinoa, which will increase your muscles' glucose levels so you can have a workout that's intense and strong the next day.

HABIT: Naturally increase your T levels daily by using the tips above.

TIP: seek medical advice if you're concerned your T levels are low. Take a few test a year to monitor the T Levels throughout the year (cost may be a factor).

SHORTCUT: There are none. It takes a month or so to feel the benefits from increased testosterone unless you're on steroids or a medically supervised testosterone enhancer.

** I have personally tried one supplement (see below) that I had seen and felt a difference (recovery). You can try it at your OWN risk. I may grow a separate limb someday, so I don't recommend this to anyone. I'm just being transparent. At forty-three years old, I was helping 2 world-class wrestlers get ready for the World Tournament and needed to increase my muscle endurance and strength as they were twenty-five and twenty-seven respectively.

Please NOTE:

- I lifted heavy to increase strength and wrestled more for endurance. I used this for a boost only.
- Taking this supplement or using any workout will not work unless you train hard and use it.

Supplement: Extreme P6 by Cellucor

BOTTOM-LINE: Try to increase your testosterone naturally. Eat lean protein, medium chain triglycerides (MCTS), complex carbs and lift heavy.

11

DIETARY ACTION NO. 11

MY TOP SHOPPING LIST TO STAY FIT

Below are the basics that have helped me stay on track to be fit and healthy.

- Low-fat cottage cheese: Daisy Brand (unless you can find a brand that's not loaded with preservatives).
- Plain, unsweetened natural Greek yogurt: add raw nuts, fresh fruit, maple syrup or natural honey (optional).
- **Unsweetened** coconut, almond, hemp, cashew, organic 2% or whole milk
- Frozen organic Fruit: blueberries, blackberries, cherries, pineapple, strawberries, mango
- Organic and/or Free Range Meats: buffalo, chicken breast and bone in, steak (sirloin), ground meats (chicken, beef, turkey)
- Fish: cod, halibut, haddock, shrimp, tuna, wild salmon, canned or packed light tuna in sunflower oil
- Sushi: fresh raw fish

- Snacks: tortillas made of brown rice, quinoa or stone ground corn. Salsa, natural hummus, organic carrots, brown rice cakes (Lundberg), stone ground quinoa and corn chips (not flour)

- Cereals: gluten free oats, steel cut oats, oat bran, quick oats, Ezekiel Cereal

- Soups: Amy's Lentil Soup (canned), Whole Foods Pre-made Chicken Soup

- Bread: Ezekiel flourless, millet bread

- Good Fats: extra virgin olive oil, raw coconut oil, Earth Balance Butter, Raw Nuts (almonds, cashews, walnuts, pistachios), raw nut butter (cashew, almond, peanut), avocado (natural guacamole)

- Seeds: chia, flax, hemp, sunflower

- Lentils

- Organic Fruit: blueberries, apples, grapefruit, pears, pineapple, watermelon, oranges, bananas

- Organic Greens: baby kale, spinach, red leaf lettuce, arugula, romaine, Swiss chard

- Complex Carbs: short grain brown rice, lentils, yams, organic potatoes (red bliss or Yukon), quinoa, barley, pasta (Tinkyada brown rice pasta made from brown rice not flour).

- Veggies: broccoli, peppers (red, yellow, orange, green), broccollini, squash, string beans, asparagus, bok choy, zucchini.

- Condiments: RAO'S pasta sauce, Newman's Own Light Dressings, natural hot sauce, organic ketchup, natural stone ground mustard, organic fruit preserve, natural maple syrup or agave, raw sugar, Braggs Liquid Amino (low sodium), garlic powder, pepper (black, cayenne, red) and salt (Himalayan or sea salt)

- Fresh herbs: parsley, basil, thyme, rosemary, garlic
- Protein powders: **natural** whey, casein, hemp, pea and/or brown rice protein. (**no** fake sugars, chemicals, anti-biotic milk sources, high salt content)

12

FOOD ACTION NO. 12

TEMPORARILY TRACK YOUR CALORIES

If you're real serious about losing weight and/or gaining muscle, then track your intake of protein, carbohydrates, fat and calories. Simply, download a food and nutrition app to help guide you. Myfitnesspal, Go Meals, Lose it are some of the apps that come to mind. Most are free, so try them out and see which one you like best. Tracking calories **should only be temporary AND not a requirement**. If you make healthy food choices and workout, then you really shouldn't bother tracking calories. Calorie tracking is important to get going with a weight loss plan, athletic performance or just for the joy of keeping numbers.

NOTE: a calorie is not just a calorie. If they were then I could eat a snickers bar worth 100 calories and skip eating 100 calories of grilled chicken. You are what you eat. **"Eat shit and you'll look like shit!"** Yes, I know. There are exceptions. You know someone who has been eating crap their entire life but still look great. Ha. Wait till their thirty or forty years old. Plus, what is their overall health? Let me change that, **"Eat shit and you'll look and feel like shit!"**

HABIT: track your meals for 2 weeks to see a pattern in your eating. Make sure to track everything you eat!

TIP: Buy a foods scale to weigh your food if you have over 20lbs. to lose and really want to keep track of your food. This will help you eye the proper portions for each food.

SHORTCUT: Work your ass off. To get fast results, train hard, eat lean and go for it.

BOTTOM-LINE: **Dietary tracking can make you more aware of what you're eating and not eating,** to reach your goal. Basically, it's scientific data to keep you accountable and on track.

13

FOOD ACTION NO. 13

LOSING WEIGHT, MINDSET AND COMMITTING

Losing weight can be tough. I get it. It takes a lot of self-control. After the age of 30, dropping pounds just gets harder and harder. I am here to tell you that if you are having a difficult time losing weight you need to change your relationship with food and workout with weights (building muscle is key). Dieting doesn't have to be just boiled chicken. Yet, you have to completely change your mindset and your relationship with food. Until you're totally sick of feeling tired, fat and just simply unhealthy. You probably won't stick to losing all your unwanted weight.

NOTE: you have to build muscle to manage your weight the best. If you don't build muscle and just lose weight. You'll be doing the typical yo-yo diet. Lose weight, eat something bad and gain weight. Adding muscle will increase your metabolism and allow you to eat a little more without the big weight swings.

Here's the Steps to use:

Say to yourself, "I'm ready to lose weight, change my eating habits and commit to it." "I can do this and will." "I'm going to use food as a fuel source and not for comfort." "I plan to lose X amount of weight in the next x weeks." (Obviously give yourself a realistic time table. Yet, push yourself to lose weight fast. Losing weight quickly will give you more motivation to keep going. Listen, I had to cut down from 155 lbs. in college to 125lbs. in a month and believe me, it wasn't easy. Yet, I had a goal and stuck to it. If needed, I could do it again.) I'm telling you, anyone can take action and lose the weight. Get tough. Take control of your body. You can do it.

Here are some important steps to take action (say these):

First: " I will eat these foods only: whole foods, lean protein, organic greens and fruit, whole grains and good fats."

Second: "I will cut down on portion sizes and fill up on greens and fresh organic fruits"

Third: "I will drink water throughout day."

Fourth: "I will become more active, workout at least 15 minutes a day with weights and will commit to moving my body every day."

HABIT: **Simply cut back on portions, eat more frequently, and eat whole foods that are natural**. Real butter, real dairy, organic meats and so on. Yes, whole food choices will cost a little more. If you have a tight budget, then search for coupons, sales, buy in bulk and freeze etc. Simply cut your portions, and your body will adjust. Fill yourself with greens rather than carbs. Eat more fruit rather than chips.

TIP: sweat your ass off (cardio at least 30 minutes every day) and train with weights (heavy and light) at least 3x per week for minimum 15 minutes. Stay on a calorie based diet and weigh your food if necessary (depends if you have to lose more than 10 lbs. and how badly you want to lose weight).

SHORTCUT: If you can't manage your diet, make it simple and stick to the same menu until you lose weight. If this doesn't work and you need more accountability then sign-up to Weight Watchers or one of these calorie type diets but use only all natural foods, scrap their premade foods.

Example:

Meal 1

- Complex Carb, Lean Protein

Meal 2

- Good Fat, Fruit

Meal 3

- Greens, Veggies, Lean Protein

Meal 4

- Good Fat, Fruit or ½ cup Low-Fat Greek Yogurt or Cottage Cheese

Meal 5

- Greens, Veggies, Lean Protein

BOTTOM-LINE: **Losing weight is not simple unless you've built up a lot of muscle in the past or you're a metabolic freak. Always eat all natural whole foods. Remove all processed foods (fast foods), refined sugars (baked goods) and fake foods (artificial sweeteners) from your diet and kitchen (do this for your family too).** Get ready to change your mindset and stay committed.

MY TOP ACTIONS TO LOSING WEIGHT

1. Sweat Your Ass Off (Fit Action # 4)
2. Workout at Least 15 Minutes (Fit Action #12)
3. Go Natural (Food Action #2)
4. Track Calories, if you have a difficult time dropping weight (Food Action #12)

14

FOOD ACTION NO. 14

KEYS TO STAYING ON A HEALTHY FOOD PLAN

Look, unless you're 18 or even in your twenties. Do you think you really have the time to worry about rotating your carbs one day, eating paleo for a month until you mess up and you gain the weight back faster then you can imagine by popping a few carbs in your mouth. Unless you want to get up on stage, a CrossFit Fanatic or walk around with your arms out to the sides, to make yourself think you're tough, but not. Fuck all that quick fix, cycling food shit. While I'm at it, screw all the guru feel good and be one with your food shit too. Nothing is better than a guru doctor telling you how to lose weight when they have a gut or they are so frail that a strong wind could throw them across the street.

If you were to ask me, **"Doug what's the best diet plan to follow?"**

For overall healthy, I'd point you towards **a Mediterranean diet** but and I repeat **but, I'd use oils sparingly.** You should be able to get enough fat in seeds, grains and simply adding a tablespoon of a high oleic oil to a salad or cooking. .

The key to staying healthy is eating all natural foods, working out every day, buying healthy condiments and finding good easy recipes. Make your diet convenient, healthy and interesting. Convenience and taste are important factors to staying on a good diet. My #1 key to eating healthy is buying premade natural foods that I can simply heat up or quickly cook and eat right away whenever needed in a pinch. This way, I don't need to eat any fast food that's loaded with fat, preservatives, sodium and so on. Plus, I enjoy what I'm eating.

Examples of what I'm referring too:

Example one: The other day I got home and brushed on garlic infused olive oil onto a bone in chicken breast. Sprinkled on some sea salt and whipped it onto the grill. While cooking, I sautéed some kale, spinach, shitake mushrooms and diced carrots in a tsp. olive oil. Heated some Trader Joes' Frozen Brown Rice and mixed that together with sautéed veggies. Once the chicken was done, I put on the plate the chicken, rice and veggies plus 2 handfuls of prewashed organic Olivia's' salad greens with organic cherry tomatoes and a little feta cheese. Topped the salad with Newman's Own Light Caesar dressing. See healthy and taste good too. Try it.

Example two: I got home on a Sunday after doing yard work for 2 hours. Took a pot, threw in a pound of organic ground beef and ¼ cup of water. Put the flame on high, covered the pan and let it cook for 8 minutes. Mashed the beef up with a fork and occasionally stirred it until all done. Once done, I let it slightly cook down and mixed in RAO'S Pasta Sauce. Placed 8-10 ounces of the beef in sauce and placed it on top of mixed greens. Lightly covered the beef with fresh parmesan cheese and done. On the side I had a large wedge of watermelon.

Now these are only a few examples, but I hope you get the drift. You can do this for any of your favorite foods. Simply, swap ingredients and make the recipe healthier. Also, make your meals easy to cook by utilizing the abundance of natural foods that are premade.

TIP: Enjoy your food. Once you reach your ideal goal weight. Create a food plan that incorporates the healthies version of your favorite foods.

HABIT: Eat all natural foods. Drink water throughout the day. Eat a variety of food.

SHORTCUT: Purchase natural, low-fat premade foods. Read labels to make sure the ingredients are natural, low-fat and low-sodium and low in refined sugars.

BOTTOM-LINE: **Keep your fridge cabinets stocked with natural premade foods to make easy and fast meals.** Choose a Mediterranean type diet to follow for a long-term healthy food plan.

*Make sure your diet is in line with any dietary medical condition you may have (diabetes, high blood pressure, high cholesterol, gluten sensitivity).

15

FOOD ACTION NO. 15

GO VEGAN OR VEGETARIAN

This could be another book. A Vegan Diet can be complicated because it takes a diet that integrates many foods to get a balanced amino acid profile while excluding all animal products including eggs and dairy. However, a vegan diet possibly can be the most nutritious and healthy diet if done correctly. I personally eat just fruits, veggies, salads, nuts, seeds and lentils for 3 days per month (void of all animal protein). After the third day, I feel great. So, try this yourself if you desire.

A vegetarian diet may be better for your lifestyle because it's less strict then a vegan diet.

Can I put on muscle if I eat a vegan or vegetarian diet?

Yes! You may not be Arnold but you certainly can be very muscular. If you're eating a vegan diet, you have to make sure you make a concerted effort to consume enough foods that will supply your body with vitamin b-12, protein, iron and calcium. Yet, a vegetarian diet will give you more than enough food options to pack on muscle.

HABIT: every month for 2 to 3 days eat a vegan type diet void of animal protein. Detox and cleanse your body.

TIP: drink lots of water. Eat fresh fruit, green juices, greens, steamed veggies, nuts, seeds, hemp protein and lentils.

SHORTCUT: discover an all-natural food store that serves an array of low-fat vegan meals to go. Whole Foods has many options.

BOTTOM-LINE: **I suggest sitting down with a nutritionist or dietician** who has a vast knowledge of a vegan or vegetarian diet. It's important that your diet doesn't lack B Vitamins, Niacin, Branched Chain Aminos and other necessary nutrients.

16

1 FOOD ACTION NO. 16

<u>ELIMINATE</u> ALL FAKE FOODS!

I saved the most important Dietary Action for last. If you use one of these tips, do your family and yourself a favor, use this one. **Absolutely eliminate all fake sugars, fats and modified foods from your diet.** These foods are chemical drugs and are horrendous and I'm shocked that so many Americans consume them like candy. I believe you're playing Russian roulette when you consume these every day. Yes, nothing may happen to you just like if you smoke cigarettes. However, you are increasing your risk for weight gain, diabetes, cancer and a host of other complications. This topic could be a book on its own.

HABIT: cut all unnatural foods from your diet.

TIP: Replace fake sugars (sucralose, Saccharin, Acesulfame Potassium, Aspartame) with one of the following: local honey, organic raw sugar, natural maple syrup, stevia, organic agave.

Replace margarines, butter sprays, etc. with one of the following: Olive Oil, Organic Butter, Earth Balance Butter, Avocado, Coconut Oil.

Replace nonfat creams, milk, etc. with one of the following: organic whole milk, unsweetened nondairy milk (hemp, cashew, almond), organic cream

SHORTCUT: Make the cut.

BOTTOM-LINE: **ELIMATE ALL FAKE FOODS FROM YOUR DIET.**

The End

So, you've made it to the end of *Fit Actions!*

Below is a reference guide that I hope will help you Take Action and reach your goal. These are the most important actions to take without getting overwhelmed. I really hope this book can help you.

Weight Loss:

- Get Ready Action 1,2,4,5
- Fitness Action 2,4,5,6,7,12,14,15,30
- Food Action 1,2,4,5,7,8,13,16

Weight Gain:

- Get Ready Action 1,2,4,5
- Fitness Action 2,4,7,8,9,10,12,13,19,25,26,27,28,29,31
- Food Action: 1,2,3,4,5,6,10,16

Get Fit and Healthy:

- Get Ready Action 1,2,4,5
- Fitness Action 1,2,3,4,6,12,15,16,18,19,30,32
- Food Action 1,2,3,6,7,8,13,14,15,16

NEED EXPERT HELP?

BOOK A CALL BY CLICKING BELOW:

COACHEDFITRX.COM

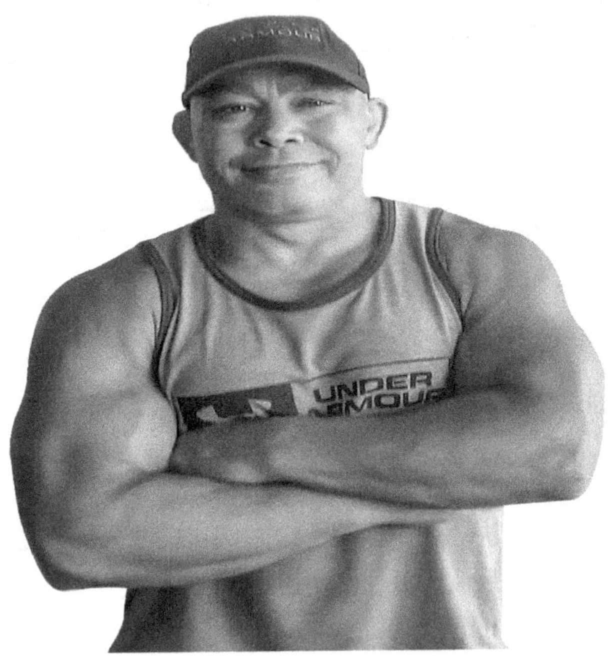

Need to ask a question or tell me to go fuck myself?

Just email me, bsstudio@comcast.net.